THE PSYCHO SQUAD

THE PSYCHO SQUAD

WILLIAM W. CRAIN, PH.D.

SATURDAY REVIEW PRESS / E.P. DUTTON & CO., INC.

NEW YORK

This book is an effort to describe the Psychiatric Emergency Team and to show how it has functioned. It is no part of our purpose to identify the individuals who have been patients or who have had to invoke the law or who have been involved in its operations. Accordingly, the names, physical descriptions, and circumstances of everyone in the book (except the author) have been changed so as to preserve their anonymity. If the names that have been used correspond to names of real people, living or dead, this is purely coincidental and unintended.

FIRST EDITION
10 9 8 7 6 5 4 3 2 1

Published simultaneously in Canada
by Clarke, Irwin & Company Limited, Toronto and Vancouver
ISBN: 0-8415-0419-9

Library of Congress Cataloging in Publication Data

Crain, William W
The psycho squad.

1. Crisis intervention (Psychiatry)—Cases, clinical reports, statistics. I. Title. [DNLM: 1. Emergency health services. 2. Mental disorders. WM100 C887p] RC480.5.C65 1976 616.8'9'025 75-29186

For Kay, and Bill and Steve

"There are no psychiatric emergencies."

(Old psychiatric saying)

ACKNOWLEDGMENT

My sincere gratitude to my editor, Milicent Tryon, for her warmth, her spirited encouragement, and her enthusiasm. She was always positive, provocative, and helpful; without her this book would not have been possible.

THE PSYCHO SQUAD

INTRODUCTION

It is becoming increasingly difficult for one to keep separate and clear his inner, subjective world from the objective world of outside events that we call external reality.

There are those among the younger generation who would claim, with the followers of Eastern religious cults, that the outside world is an illusion. The real world is inside, within the inner space of our psyches. The media, and our profound dependence upon them, haven't helped matters. That intimate stranger, television, has moved into our homes as a permanent guest with all its involving, intoxicating goings-on. We talk back to the set like little children and root aloud for the home team as if we were there in the stands.

To add to our disorientation, we have experienced a distinct loss of faith in leaders and other "example" figures. We are confused as to the reality, the sincerity, of an individual's words and outward actions as they might provide valid evidence of what the person is really like. Leaders deliberately seek to have a "positive image." But are a leader's actions "him," or are they put-ons, like a suit of clothes donned in the morning to face the day and fool the people? Just as the media present us with actors pretending to be real, so we may wonder if "real" people are in fact acting.

If the average person, coming from a reasonably stable home environment, is confused, the reader may imagine what it is like for one whose hold on reality has always been tenuous.

We will meet some of these people in this book. They appear bewildered, trying desperately to find footing in a slippery, chimerical world, a now-you-see-it, now-you-don't reality of a Vietnam that probably never happened, of a future shock that is passé.

More significantly, these individuals do not know *where* they are. In these stories of people encountered by the Psychiatric Emergency Team, (whose names have been changed) I have attempted to capture the feeling of those who seem to be the real victims of this confusing, anchorless world of overlapping realities.

The emergency team frequently encounters people standing on the brink of madness. And, because we see them on the home front, we see their families, and sense the interaction, the way it was between them, before this particular member lost hold and fell into madness. For madness is a *place.* It is a world, another world. Another of those alternatives so popular these days.

The assignment is ambiguous, confusing. Going *out* into the community—right into homes, "invited" by someone who may or may not know what he is doing when he opens the door to us—does not always make a lot of sense. Yet something has to be done. Relatives, parents, everyone involved is at wit's end. Maybe the police have been called. They leave, doing nothing. "It's a mental case," they say. They give them our number.

The Lanterman-Petris-Short Act in California permits certain designated professionals—psychiatrists, psychologists, psychiatric social workers, and psychiatric nurses—to sign an individual into the hospital for a period of seventy-two hours *involuntarily* if, in the judgment of those professionals, the person is a danger to himself, a danger to others, or gravely disabled. Once hospitalized, he can be detained in the hospital without his consent, following psychiatric and court review.

It is a potentially controversial law, though there has been little controversy surrounding it. PET teams are cropping up in many of the major cities of the United States. We positively love innovation and novelty in this country, and PET is the latest thing.

People have been picked up as "psychos" for many years now. The laws of past years permitted relatives, police officers, wives and husbands, even business partners, to be involved in the certification that a person was insane. Who can doubt that the wrong person occasionally was sent away? Then followed that nightmare of nightmares, being detained in the hospital until one agreed that one was indeed mentally ill and needed the treatment that was being offered, such as it was. The new laws protect, that is true. There are all manner of built-in safeguards. But the primary protection of the "innocent" or sane citizen is that it is expensive to maintain large institutions.

By tradition, clinicians located themselves in some set place at some set time. The "patient" or "client" would bring himself in to see someone, or a parent or relative brought him. Now things are different. Just as people may be "acting out" in increasing degree, so is our act "out" in that place called the "community." We are the latest thing in white coats and butterfly nets. We enter homes, we evaluate, and we scoop up.

Typically we work in pairs on the emergency team, much like the police. The two professionals who respond to a call include a clinician (social worker, psychologist, or psychiatrist) and a psychiatric technician with experience in the state hospitals. My partner most of the time was a calm, older psych tech whom I will call Harry Barnes.

Frequently the patient has been hospitalized previously. Without intending a criticism of the dedicated and hard working staff in California's state and/or private hospitals, the mere threat of reinstitutionalization is enough to jar many of these people. Out of contact as they may be, we sometimes threaten them with such action to get them to conform to "reality" and to take the medication they have been neglecting.

Professionals who find themselves on emergency assignment may agree that there are few options available in most cases. It is temporary hospitalization or further regression, and nothing in between. Left to his own pitiful resources, the typical person in deep emotional trouble may actually die of malnutrition. He may walk in front of a car. He may kill himself. Occasionally—this is a rare occurrence—he may hurt or kill somebody else.

What about the person's civil rights? I believe this entire question can stand an airing before PET teams become a fixture everywhere. Isn't it an invasion of privacy for a clinician to knock on a door and introduce himself as a professional seeking to "evaluate" a person? Wouldn't many of us do a lot of wondering about ourselves for the next few weeks if approached this way? Wouldn't we become a bit paranoid? Watchful of our friends and relatives? Surely some open-minded readers will discover a few of their many selves within these pages.

One can view the problem of the civil rights of the individual in the abstract and the general sense. The abuses of the CIA and the FBI are examples of violations which affect all of us, at least indirectly. This narrative looks at the individual case and may bring the problem closer to home.

Maybe that critical social problem—the protection of an individual's right to privacy—is nowhere better illuminated than in these true-life situations where the agents are standing on the person's doorstep, knocking on his door.

This is an accounting of my own involvement in emergency activity roughly spanning the period from November 1972, when I first joined the PET team, to January 1974.

1

The beginnings were instructive if inauspicious for the Psychiatric Emergency Team, West Valley Section. Other regional offices had begun their PET services earlier, but they were located in the central city. This was still country in the spring of 1970, here on the edge of Los Angeles County's gigantic sprawl. Ventura County is a short distance to the west. The Pacific Ocean is twelve miles or so over the hill toward Malibu.

West Valley's PET team had three eager members—a nurse, a psychiatric technician, and a psychologist. They had been called to evaluate an elderly lady who was bothering passers-by at a nearby shopping center.

"Is this the Mental Health Service?"

"Yes."

"Are you the guys with the butterfly nets?"

"Look, we don't consider . . ." This was serious business and the team was nervous.

"I know. I was kidding. There is this old lady over here in the parking lot. She is really out of her tree. She stops people and lectures them about the coming end of the world. It's a real downer, for one thing."

"This doesn't sound like a case for our office. She doesn't

sound as though she would qualify as a danger to self or others. And we require real evidence, you know."

"It's not enough to be a real nut?"

"We don't call people nuts, you know."

"OK, have it your way. She's really out of it, though. Are you just going to let this lady wander around like this?"

The team talked it over. They didn't know what they were doing, really. The new Lanterman-Petris-Short Act was ambiguous to say the least. Too much room for interpretation, even though it focused on behavior, not insanity. How much of a danger was this lady? Not likely a danger to others. Possibly to self. Was she eating, for instance? The young man was smart. He was leaving it up to them. They had pictures of a helpless, psychotic old lady starving to death out in that desert of anonymity, a West Valley shopping center.

"She's wearing a transparent raincoat," the young man said. "And she's carrying an open umbrella."

"So?"

"It's not raining."

"We know. So she's a little bit off. We don't hospitalize people merely because they're considered crazy, you know. Anyway, if we hospitalize her, we're only empowered to sign her in for seventy-two hours. They'll probably release her from Camarillo in three days."

"If you saw her you would hospitalize her," he said. "But have it your way." He hung up.

The PET team spotted the elderly lady in the parking lot as they drove up. She was jabbering away in front of a small crowd. As they approached, they could see that the young man had neglected to mention the old lady was *naked* beneath that transparent raincoat. Did public exposure of this old, gnarled body constitute a danger to others, let alone to the woman herself? The team, conscientious and literal as people will be on new assignments, decided to review the alternatives.

"She's not a *danger* to anybody. She's helpless. She doesn't know what she's doing."

"She's waving that umbrella around, and she'll stick somebody."

"She's bothering people."

"Did you ever see such wrinkled boobs? We had better call Shaefer Ambulance. Who's got their number?"

"You mean you didn't bring the briefcase? We don't have the number? What if we have to restrain her?"

The lady herself expressed curiosity at the odd little group of people standing next to the county station wagon talking away. She approached them.

"Hello there," she said. "Isn't it a nice day?"

The nurse looked up. "Yes, it is." She spoke for the group, as she was the one with real-life experience, having sped through the streets of New York in the old days.

"Could I ask you a personal question?" the nurse said.

"Oh, I don't know about that," the old lady said shrewdly. "I don't know about that."

"I was wondering why you're wearing a raincoat. And the umbrella . . . ?"

"When it begins to rain," she said loudly, turning to the small gathering, "I don't want to be caught unawares."

"Speaking of unawares," the nurse said, "are you aware of the fact that you're *naked* underneath that raincoat?"

"Of course," the lady said, "I am well aware of my present state of undress. I intend to meet my maker in the same fashion as I entered this world."

"In a plastic raincoat?"

She ignored that one and turned to her audience. "The world is coming to an end!" she shouted. "Beware! Beware!" She held the umbrella over her head. "It could rain at any moment," she said.

More reconnoitering. So what should they *do?* Was she a danger to self or others? Gravely disabled? But what exactly did that particular category refer to? Someone suggested they check on her orientation in space and time. Maybe if she were totally confused they could justify hospitalization and at least do something definite.

The nurse approached her. "I wonder if you would tell me where you live."

"Certainly."

"Well . . . where?"

"Nearby," she said coyly. "In a house."

"Could I get the address?"

"No." She turned to the bystanders. "You see, that is my own business, as you know. I am a citizen of the United States. I therefore am not required to tell *anybody* the address of my house."

The nurse looked at the psychologist. He shrugged. The crowd was beginning to understand the dilemma. The team retreated for a final huddle. She was psychotic, but see-through raincoats weren't one of the problems on the chart. She was within her rights, withholding her address. "Where are you headed?" the nurse asked her.

"I'm going shopping, dear," she said. "That's why I am here, in the shopping center."

"Of course," the nurse said.

So on their first case the PET team let the subject go. She walked off, twirling her umbrella and swinging her ancient rear provocatively. She was last observed entering a department store. She has not been reported again. Somewhere in the vast expanse of the San Fernando Valley wanders a naked old lady in a transparent raincoat who is probably quite mad. But she doesn't meet the criteria to be locked up. And it is just as well.

2

The Psychiatric Emergency Team is Harry Barnes's full-time assignment. As the clinic's psychiatric technician he will coordinate the team's activities. The rest of us have been assigned a single PET day. Mine is Friday. We are required to keep our emergency day clear of other clinic activities. If the day is quiet, we sit, like firemen, performing minor housekeeping chores, bringing records up to date, making entries into case files.

Harry Barnes is a tall, muscular black man in his early forties. He has the graceful, easy moves of a natural athlete. There is a slight, mischievous smile on his handsome face, as if he knows something the rest of us don't know. He appears absolutely unruffable. I have noted that he sometimes shows anger for the effect of it—to alter the mood of a situation to suit himself. Obviously Harry Barnes knows what he is about, even though he is as new to the clinic as I am. His presence here has had an altogether calming effect on all of us.

The newer members of the staff kid him—manipulatively—about his obvious physical strength. "You take the lead, Harry," we say. "You run the interference, OK?" He shrugs and smiles his mild, confident smile. "Sure," he says. "You decide whether they go to the hospital. I'll take care of the rest of it."

I watched Harry as he carefully arranged the contents of

the PET attaché case—the various forms we complete, sign, and hand over to the ambulance attendants who would transport the particular individual to the state hospital. The forms require a description of the reason for hospitalization and the emotional state in which the person was found. A clinician's signature permits the individual's detention in a designated psychiatric setting for seventy-two hours, not counting the weekend. He can be detained for a total of thirty days, depending upon subsequent psychiatric review. It is a power that should not be taken lightly, yet I realize even now that I will be signing those forms routinely, making diagnostic impressions that become as fixed to the person as a tattoo on his forehead.

Harry handled several bottles of tranquilizers, placing them neatly into a pocket of the case. He picked up the syringe used by the psychiatrist on emergency assignment when a patient loses control or is actively psychotic. He fingered the plastic restraints, the thin, transparent handcuffs that can be quickly fitted through a buckle to bind the patient's hands or legs. They can be removed only by cutting.

The telephone rang. Harry grabbed a four-by-seven PET card and began writing.

"Yes . . . I see . . . Is he a big boy? How old did you say?" He gave me a meaningful glance. Evidently a home visit was developing. "Are there any dangerous weapons? Any guns?" I swallowed. "Knives? All right, it sounds like a legitimate call, lady. Who referred you to this office? Yes . . . yes, lady . . ." He sighed. She talked on. Finally he obtained the cross streets near the woman's home so we could locate the place quickly on the area map of the valley on the wall behind him. Harry put down the telephone and looked at me inquiringly.

"I think we're going to have to go out on this call. It could be a rough one, Doc."

So my time had come. Why had I accepted this job in the first place? I liked the idea, the sound of it, "working out in the community." "It's where the action is," the chief psychiatrist had said when he appraised me during the hiring interview.

"You get your hands dirty on this job," he said, smiling slightly. Was it the challenge of it all? It would be something different, surely. "Sometimes, you know, we have to grab a leg, and we work closely with the police . . ." "Well," I said, "sure. Why not? I can handle it." At the same time I wondered why I was saying the words. And until that moment the last thing in the world I would have pictured myself doing was working closely with the police.

Would I be able to function in the kinds of situations I'd heard described? I thought of my past experience working with delinquents who were acting out. Well, their impulsiveness hadn't bugged me particularly, and more than once I had entered a room in the old detention unit to find a young adolescent screaming and out of control. But all I had ever done was talk. There had been others around to do the grabbing. Maybe it would be like mixing it up in half-court basketball. Jesus, I hadn't been in a physical fight since grammar school.

I approached Harry. "You know I don't approve of mistreating . . . of being overly physical, Harry," I said.

"I know, Doc," he said softly. "I know. But we got to contain them. And if the person cannot control himself . . ."

It was the old correctional jargon again: "If the boy cannot control himself, then it is necessary to control him—for his own sense of security . . ."

"What we do, Doc, is more or less lean on the person. We bring in enough bodies to weigh him down. Anyway, old Harry here has the moves, Doc, the *moves.*" He grabbed me suddenly, twisting an arm behind my back. I was completely helpless.

"OK," I said. "But I'm going to try to talk this guy into going voluntarily, like the book says. You can let loose now."

"Sure, Doc," he said. He handed me the PET telephone card. The mother of a nineteen-year-old boy had called. She was afraid he would rape her, she said. He claimed to be the anti-Christ. They were Jewish, but he was a member of a Jesus group. Last Christmas the family had squabbled over his insistence that they celebrate the holiday with a Christmas tree. Things had gone downhill since. She suspected drugs. Right at this moment he was hiding in his room. There were no weapons. She said he was small and skinny—that was part of his problem. He had a very large inferiority complex due to his small organ and had never been right since entering puberty.

We pulled the big station wagon in front of a small stucco duplex and knocked on the door. A little, round-faced lady opened the door and stared at me uncomprehendingly.

I showed her my ID.* "We're from the County Department of Mental Health . . ."

"What?" She appeared dazed.

"Is something wrong?"

"No, come on in," she said. "You'll have to excuse me. I've been under a strain."

The small living room had a barren, unlived-in feeling. A gas log burned in the fake fireplace. A strange plastic lamp stood on an end table next to the couch. Three shiny golden birds were propelled by the heat from the lamp around a plastic tree.

"Nice," Harry said.

The lady's eyes seemed filmed over, unseeing. "I haven't slept too well lately. My son Martin has been acting . . . strange. I'm not sure if he wants to harm me in some way or whether . . . you know, this sex business. It's entirely too permissive, all of this sex business."

Her tone was bland, as if she were talking about someone else. "It's not easy, you know, raising a young man in these times. My husband died seven years ago."

We knocked on the bedroom door. No answer. We knocked again. Still no answer.

"Martin!" she yelled suddenly. "You get your butt out here right now."

*"Pursuant to Section 5150, California Welfare and Institution Code, the bearer of this card has been designated by the Board of Supervisors of Los Angeles County as a professional person who upon reasonable cause may take, or cause to be taken, into custody any person who is dangerous to himself or others or gravely disabled as a result of mental disorder and place him in a treatment facility designated by the county and approved by the State Department of Mental Hygiene."

We heard a moan as if someone were in great pain. Or maybe it was a ghost and the room was haunted.

"Do you think he's all right?" I asked.

"Yes. He's just hiding. He hides during the day. He only comes out at night. Martin!"

Still no answer. Cautiously, I opened the door and looked in. No Martin. We walked in. Martin evidently enjoyed the way water worked. A large, fancy aquarium on his desk bubbled away. There were colorful, energetic little fish swimming around.

"Martin?" I said.

"Sometimes he hides in the closet," she said.

Harry slowly opened the closet door. No Martin.

"Sometimes he hides under the bed."

I slowly pulled the bedspread upward. It was dark. No Martin. Where was Martin?

"Sometimes," she said, "he crawls under the window there."

"Oh boy," Harry said. "Swell. Then you mean he just takes off? Couldn't you have made sure he was home before we drove halfway across the valley?"

Harry opened the window and leaned out.

"Boo," Martin said.

"Come on in, Martin," he said.

Martin crawled in the window. "Hi," he said. "How's it going?"

"Swell," Harry said. "Things are going really well, Martin."

We sat on the bed and talked. Martin was crazy enough, I decided, but not insane. He said calmly that he had no intention of harming anybody, not even his mother. She was the crazy one, he said. He thought it was ridiculous, absolutely ridiculous, the idea of his wanting to . . . Wow!

He seemed intact enough to tell a coherent story. We told his mother we could not hospitalize Martin. It wouldn't do a whole lot for his conception of himself. Adolescents were extremely sensitive to labels, I said. The label of mentally ill would affect him very negatively. And he clearly wasn't a danger to himself or others.

"So you are going to let him stay here and rape me. Is that the situation? Am I hearing you correctly?"

"No," I said. "It's just that . . ."

"Well, if he rapes me in the night, or kills me, like hitting me with some weapon, or stabs me in the chest with a knife while I am deep in sleep, then the blood is on your hands . . ."

Martin shuffled his feet anxiously.

We discussed placement out of the home. I talked for a time about the problems of a mother living with a grown son, without a father to help reduce the tension between them. I told her of the natural feelings between people, of the danger of too much emotion. She didn't hear a word I said.

I told Martin he had better begin making plans to leave. It was time to begin breaking the old umbilical.

"Where will I *go?*" he asked. "I want to get out of here, but I'm scared. Where would I go?"

She turned to me. "If you don't take him away, something terrible is going to happen." Words said blandly. The lady was a bystander to her own life.

Martin wiped the sweat from his forehead with his sleeve. He shifted his feet as if he were marching in place in slow motion. He looked to his mother. She was his only ally in the world, this familiar enemy who stared in his direction now as if he did not exist.

"Well, we aren't going to hospitalize your son," I said, grabbing the attaché case.

She smiled knowingly as we walked out of Martin's room. Harry stopped beside the large, colorful, bubbling aquarium. He put his face close to the water, watching the little fish swimming about.

"Martin?" he said. "Anybody seen Martin?"

* *

Harry guided the station wagon into the clinic parking area behind a tall, modern office building. The sun reflected on the black glass exterior.

"Did you get the impression that that crazy lady *wants* her son to do her in?" he asked.

"Yes, I think so," I said.

We talked about the old problem of identifying who was mad and who was sane, and how the sane ones sometimes were locked up while the insane ones made the complaint and remained free. Under the old laws this happened more frequently than one cared to think. The psychiatric evaluations weren't overly thorough, and the court had a direct hand in it all—not that a judge was adequately trained to determine mental health.

The new law emphasized *behavior.* It stressed outside, observable responses, rather than speculation regarding inner mental state. What counted, presumably, was whether a person could control himself or not, whether he was a danger to others or himself, whether he was "gravely disabled" due to an emotional disorder—all in our view.

"So it is all right to be crazy in the old sense of the word," I said, "as long as you take care of yourself and don't harm other people."

"That's an improvement, I guess," Harry said. "What it means is we are going to do an awful lot of walking away from situations like this last one, right? Even when we have a hunch that a crazy lady is going to work it out so she gets herself killed by her own son . . ."

"In her own way she was telling us what she was up to, Harry," I said, "with all of that 'my blood is on your hands' crap."

We felt we had acted appropriately on this case. We decided there was nothing to be done, except to feel vaguely guilty about it. And be especially careful not to read the newspapers.

*   *

We walked back into the PET room. Al Johnson, the young psychiatric social worker, was there. "This job keeps your adrenalin pumping," Al said, looking at us. A tall, thin young man fresh from social work field placement, he had been out on several calls already. His last call had been a messy one involving the police.

He turned to Harry. "Harry makes it easy," he said admiringly. He and Harry, accompanied by two police officers, had once subdued a middle-aged executive who was threatening to burn his house down. He was seeing things and hearing voices that told him to get rid of all his possessions.

My mouth tasted chalky. Were *all* these calls going to be this nerve-wracking?

"What they wanted to do was deck the guy," he continued. "That's how they handle their fear. But Harry here, he controlled it beautifully."

Harry had calmly and determinedly taken control of the situation, he said, placing the police in the role of "backup."

A lot of aspects of the PET assignment had never been worked out.

"One real problem is coordinating," Al said. "We didn't know, for instance, if we would have to hospitalize this guy until I evaluated him. So we had to call the ambulance from the man's house. Those bastards said they would be right over, but they didn't show for forty-five minutes. Ever try to talk that long to an insane ex-executive? Mostly he told us what a big shot he had been before he realized he would have to do away with all this phony materialism of his."

The law required a first-hand evaluation. We couldn't take anybody's word for the person's mental state. That meant we were stuck with this situation of waiting for the ambulance while trying to explain to a highly disturbed person why we were in his home territory with two or more police officers, not meaning him any particular harm.

Al had tried for thirty minutes to talk the man into allowing them to bind his wrists with the thin plastic restraints, but he refused. He began insisting and the man got increasingly agitated, talking to himself louder and louder. Then he screamed "No! No!" and suddenly rushed at one of the cops.

"I saw the cop's eyes," Al said. "He was absolutely terrified. So of course everyone jumped on the man. Including me." He shook his head sadly. "It really wasn't too cool. But you should have seen Harry. All the time the man was screaming and we were grabbing his arms and legs, old Harry was tying him up with the plastic restraints, actually calming the man down."

He licked his dry lips. "It's a long way from the USC School of Social Welfare, I'll tell you."

"Tell me about it," Harry said.

3

Another Friday. Christmas has finally passed and the new year is upon us. The air is clear and nippy outside and people move a little faster. There is a major construction project going on across the street from the PET room. I can hear the dull thud of jackhammers through the soundproofed windows. "We are having twins," the big sign says opposite. They are making two movie theaters out of one.

The holidays have been difficult. So many unhappy, unloved people contacted us in the last month or so. The spirit of Christmas reminds many people of what they never had, how things cannot substitute for love. And they feel gypped, these collectors of injustices. They somehow believe it is possible to go back into time and right past wrongs.

It is PET day for me. Oddly enough, I find that I enjoy this assignment in the main. Is it the unpredictability? The unknown? Maybe I have more cop in me than I care to acknowledge.

Several weeks have passed without a major PET call. It is odd how the telephone will ring all day long on one Friday and be almost mute the next, as if emotional disturbances follow rhythms and cycles unknown to us. Maybe there really is something to madness being influenced by the moon.

This assignment offers an intriguing view of America in action. Are we working in a kind of *living theater,* going out like this into the community? Is America deeply caught up in some theatrical madness, living out its own myth in some strange, almost self-conscious way? Are we ourselves "acting" in appropriate and official roles, or are we "acting out" in the manner of clinicians become policemen without clear restraints and time-worked role behaviors?

Harry has just taken a call from a young veteran's wife. Her husband was acting crazy, she said. He had not been himself since he had returned home from Vietnam. He was using hard drugs, and he was threatening to kill her. He had a gun.

Harry headed the big station wagon toward the middle valley area. Traces of Christmas were still in evidence on Van Nuys Boulevard. Lights were strung along porch eaves. Signs on storefronts still told of Xmas bargains.

"This sounds like a bad one," I said, just to say something. "I'm kind of nervous. Are you scared?"

"No, are you?"

"I told you I was. You must be scared or you would have heard me."

"Detach yourself, Doc," Harry said. "That's how you should handle it."

"How do you handle it?"

"I dribble in my pants."

I saw a little dog rolling in the grass. I was sad, overcome by a surge of emotion. It seemed to me that what I needed was a whole lot more of these perfect little scenes of small dogs at play.

"I'm sure the cops will move in first this time," I said. "To tell you the truth, Harry, I'm tired of all this machismo shit. I don't have anything to prove anymore. What I am is chicken-shit. That's my diagnosis. You can take this community psychiatry and shove it up your ass."

"Not my ass, Doc," he said. "How come you are so worked up?"

"Hell, I don't know. Maybe I have a premonition about this call."

The police were on the scene when we arrived. Three officers, all young, stood quietly, maintaining their cool cop look. The sergeant was a big, friendly man with a bushy mustache and bulging gut. A beer drinker.

"So what's the plan?" Sarge spoke with a mildly sarcastic twang. "I hear there may be a gun."

"There is a gun," I said. "That's what the wife said on the phone. She said your department was here last night but you took off without doing anything."

"I know," he said. I had irritated him. Never tell a policeman anything directly. He will check the sky for falling bird droppings. "So what should we do?" he asked. "It's your show."

I glanced at Harry. It was "our show." Now we had to watch for the PD quick step. How were we going to get the police to take the lead with a cool sergeant like this one? The officers stood as if nailed. Nobody moved.

Sarge's eyes narrowed in on me. He was checking me for signs of chickenheartedness.

Harry moved in. "Look, this is how we are going to work it. You guys—you knock on the door. You take the lead . . ." He cleared his throat. "You guys make sure there is no gun. Or you get the gun . . . you know . . . and then we'll . . ."

"Look," the sergeant said, irritated. "We can't just *knock* on the fucking *door,* in full *view* like that. If this turkey has a fucking *piece,* and he says he's going to *use* it, well, crap, I can't ask my men to just walk up and knock on the fucking *door.*"

"Well," I said, "maybe you could just stand back . . ."

"Would *you* want to take a fucking chance like that? Goddamn, Doctor, I can't just send my men in like that. Maybe we should get the gun squad out here. We can line up a fucking army, you know. We'll get that fucking piece. I'm going to . . ." He moved to the side as if he were going to make the call.

"No," I said, "I know he has a gun in there, but we don't know if it's loaded. His wife said he is probably asleep . . ." I wanted to get it over with.

"Well, if he's sleeping, where is the wife?"

"She said she would be in there," I told him.

"Crap," Harry said, "I'm going to knock on the door."

"We'll be right here," Sarge said. "We'll back you up. You can rely on us. I mean it." He winked at me.

"Fucker," I said.

He heard me. "Now is that a way for a doctor to talk?" he said, smiling widely. Somehow I had risen in his estimation.

Harry and I walked up to the apartment. It looked like nobody was home. We knocked.

Harry knocked again, loudly. No sounds from inside. "Hey!" he shouted. "Anybody home?" No answer. The tension mounted. I looked down. Sarge was leaning against the wall. His eyes were closed. A cigarette hung loosely from his mouth.

"Well," I said, "nobody home. Let's split."

We were both thinking the same thing. What if everybody inside was dead? Harry looked ashen. He hit his head hard with his hand.

"What's wrong?" I said.

"Doc, this isn't B-310; it's A-310. We got the wrong apartment."

It was Sarge's idea at that point to break for lunch. "Look," he said, "there really isn't any big hurry with this psycho, right? Let's have some lunch. My men are all worked up. We could use a break."

We stood around together for a few moments, embarrassed. "Let's meet back here at exactly one o'clock, OK?" Harry said.

We split up. At lunch Harry and I discussed policemen and their psychology. We agreed we might be encountering a new breed, or maybe they were covering themselves better. I told him about a recent ticket for speeding, how I tried to get the fact that I worked with policemen into the conversation.

I told him about a young policeman who had brought in a disturbed woman the week previously. He had bragged about outsmarting the psychologist who evaluated all the new recruits. He said he really outfoxed him on the Rorschach. "You know, that card where there's a big gorilla with a cock a foot long?" he said. "I told him it was a crazy motorcyclist driving a hundred miles an hour down the freeway. Wouldn't catch me telling that shrink about all those cocks and pussies on those cards." He had passed the tests.

Lunch had to end. We met the three policemen down the street crouched behind some massive hedges. We approached apartment B-310. Through the screen door I saw the bottoms of a man's feet. He was lying on the couch. That meant he was asleep. Or resting. Or training a loaded gun on the doorway. I figured I had faced death once already that day so somehow this second time didn't count. In the shuffle for position Harry ended up in the lead. I walked in behind him.

The young veteran was sprawled on the couch sound asleep. His pretty young wife greeted us with a smile. She turned her eyes to her husband. He leaped up, startled, as if he had felt her gaze. He lurched toward us.

"What the hell!" he said. "This is my house, man. You can't come barging in here."

"Sit down, asshole," Sarge's voice came booming in. "Sit down or I'll play a tune on your fucking gourd. This here is a *doctor.* He wants to talk to you. He wants to see if you're all right in your fucking *head.* You cooperate, you hear." He twirled his baton for effect. It stuck out menacingly like a twelve-inch erection.

The young vet decided to make a show of protest. "You have no right to come in here . . ."

"We were called in," I said.

"By who? By who?" Now he was near tears. There were dark circles under his eyes from weeks of sleeplessness. He scanned the room, checking his chances.

"We hear you have a gun," I said.

He ignored me. He threw his hands to the side in a gesture of surrender and turned to his pretty wife. "You?" he screamed. "You called them. You're really out to fuck me. You really mean to do it." He seemed amazed, almost respectful.

She smiled at him. She had become the center of attention. Sarge examined her closely, his eyes glassy with lust. Her husband stared at her, bewildered. She appeared excited, as if she were enjoying the drama. She returned Sarge's stare, forcing him to drop his eyes.

"Man, I've been had, you know," the vet was saying to a policeman. "I have really been had." He hung his head. He addressed the rug. "Who *are* you guys, anyway?"

She turned from him as if he didn't exist. Sarge made his play. "Pal, we hear you got a piece. We hear you have been making fucking threats to kill people. How about that?" He waved his baton again.

Harry spoke up. "We have this complaint. All we want to do is talk to you, to make an evaluation."

"Talk to them, baby," she said, looking at Harry. "They only want to help you."

"Why would I want to kill anybody?" he shouted. "I don't have a gun. Who called you? What are you doing here?" He held his hand on his forehead. "I don't feel too good." He sat down on the couch and mumbled to himself.

His wife caught Sarge's eye. "Son of a bitch is really out of it," he said. "You better call the ambulance."

I stalled. "Has he been on dope?" I asked.

She nodded.

The young vet awakened from his daydreams. "How come I have to be the patsy for all this?" he asked, whining. "Did she call you guys? How come I got to be the fall guy?"

"Where's the gun?" Harry asked.

"I don't have a gun. I just said I had a gun, but I don't."

I turned to the young woman. She shrugged. She beckoned softly to Sarge. They whispered in the corner.

Sarge walked over to Harry and me. "There isn't any gun," he said. "She says she was afraid we wouldn't come if she didn't say he had a gun and was dangerous. I can understand. . . . Aren't you going to call the ambulance?"

The vet was busy talking to himself. He had that flushed, little-kid look on his face.

"Have you ever been busted?" I asked the vet.

He looked up. "Yeah. Yeah, I was in the Youth Authority. Why?"

"Just the way you looked. I don't know. What's going on here?"

He shrugged. "This is a secret opium den." He examined the floor. "I need help, I guess. I'm really all fucked up in the head. I think I'm going crazy."

He screamed at the men in white from Shaefer as they entered the room. He had changed his mind. A crowd gathered outside. He laughed hysterically as they bound him to the gurney. He offered no real opposition so they used the soft cloth restraints.

Later as we drove off Harry asked me if I had noticed the girl's eyes. I hadn't.

"Dilated pupils, Doc," he said. "Probably really was an opium den. Heroin, anyway. Why do you suppose she wanted him out of there?"

We were again wondering if we had sent off the wrong one. We had come in at the end of this movie and there were so many loose ends, so many things we would never know.

4

Friday is the busiest day for emotional crises in the San Fernando Valley. Anticipation of the weekend heightens anxieties. Family members are forced together, adding to existing tensions. People who are depressed or extremely lonely dread the weekends. They are faced with themselves, with their feelings of rejection and isolation. Can't even lose themselves in their work roles.

The experience of inner emptiness can be terrifying, frantic. Community help lines, suicide prevention, and the PET are all jumping on the weekends. The secretary there, filing your files, seriously considered ending it all last weekend.

The boss there, smiling his big, confident smile, cried like a baby Saturday night. He begged his mistress not to leave him and crawled, actually crawled, at her feet. She refused him. He got angry as hell and he roared on homeward, hoping the cars in the opposite lane would jump the divider. His hands held tightly to the wheel. Should he turn it now? He managed to drag himself to work the next day. At the door of the building he put on his familiar mask, ready to gut it out. If he doesn't let down and admit at some point that he isn't superman, he won't make it to fifty.

So many despairing people. They call the clinic. The intake worker tries to make an appointment in a day, a week from now, depending on the backload of cases. Some cannot wait. People hold on, hold on—until they crack.

We are having a run of the strangest telephone calls. A young man describes his hangup with masturbation. He becomes increasingly explicit. There are giggles in the background. He is putting us on. Entertaining his friends. The question is, does he really have the problem he is kidding about? A mother calls. Her son is acting odd. She spends twenty minutes telling us what a good mother she has been. We learn not to ask the obvious questions. Fiercely angry people tell us off, demand immediate action, seek to have us do their parental job for them. We learn to let them drain the anger off. Don't respond or argue. So many people simply want to be *heard.* We learn to catch the tone of voice that says this is a serious case.

I talk to a woman who says she has taken some pills. Could she make it in to the clinic? Could she take a taxi? Yes? Well, come on in. She arrives, miraculously, weaving drunkenly through the lobby, half dead. Wrong move that time.

We are firemen, mental health firemen, on emergency day, putting out fires. Much of the time we are bluffing and faking. Do this, do that. It seems to work. They don't call back, anyway.

Terrible, awful, impossible problems, not acted upon. Do they simply disappear? Not always, but sometimes they seem to. Like ignoring a metallic sound in your car motor. It goes away once in a while. What happened to that woman who thought her husband was going to kill her? What about that man who was flipping out? Home visits not made due to limited staff. Nothing more is heard. Better not read the newspapers too closely.

An acquaintance, every time he sees me, asks, "How are your nuts?" I am not sure which nuts he is referring to. Fine, I want to say. How are yours? He, like many other people, assumes that madness happens to somebody else. Somebody weak, basically. To some, it is almost un-American to break down.

*　　　　*

I looked across my desk at a handsome older man—"Mr. Edward Sherwin," the PET card said, "age 52." He didn't look the type to be in a clinic like this. He wore an expensive suit and a fifteen-dollar tie. Mr. Sherwin, I said to myself, you are too distinguished-looking to be in mental trouble. You should be more bedraggled.

The card said he had lost his job in recent months. How many more of you will take this particular way out, Mr. Sherwin? Does it beat jumping off a bridge?

He sat quietly across from me. He was polite. His brow was permanently furrowed so his worries flowed freely around his forehead. I looked at him and thought, Mr. Sherwin, you are a runaway, that's what you are. Sure you are hurting in there. But where you are now is no picnic, right? Was that a slight nod?

He shuffled his feet, rose and offered a big, thick hand to me. I shook it.

"How *are* you?" he said, as if it were now time for us to meet. He was deeply interested in my welfare. Had we met before? He looked familiar.

"I'm fine," I said. "I'm Dr. Crain."

"Are you now? That's nice. So then it's hello Dr. Crain, isn't it? It is a pleasure to meet you, Dr. Crain. A genuine pleasure." Dale Carnegie phrases, always sadly said. They hang out there in public, naked and unprotected. Are you the same man, Mr. Sherwin, that I was twenty years ago, made so wretched by the Carnegie course? He faced me heroically, maintaining eye contact like you were supposed to. He thought people were out to kill him but he forced himself to look at them anyway, friendly like.

"Do you have any idea why these policemen brought you here to the clinic, Mr. Sherwin?"

"Of course I do, Doctor. Of course I do." He was puzzled. "It was their opinion, Doctor, that I was behaving in a way not conducive. They have every right to believe that. Not that it is up to me, in a manner of speaking, to give them, or you, or anybody, for that matter, the right to their opinion. It is . . ."

The old obsessiveness, the old doubt. The old rigid, well-worn phrases flowed unchecked now on rusty old tracks. Weeds all around. The old engine puffed along toward Right Knowledge, but it was miles past and years ago and no way to turn back.

"Mr. Sherwin, the officers tell us that you were standing on the street corner, more or less harassing people walking by. The women, especially."

"No, that is not an accurate designation of the situation. No, that is not what would be termed an accurate or even precise or, for that matter, truly concise appraisal of the situation."

I studied Mr. Sherwin. What were you like as a kid, Mr. Sherwin? Did the company realize what it was doing when it let you go, Mr. Sherwin? That was probably how they said it to you: "Sorry, Sherwin, but we have to let you go." Did they know how accurately the phrase described the process, "letting Sherwin go"?

He began speaking. "They say I am crazy. I got fired. Did you know there was a fire?"

"Yes," I said. I know about that. When you get fired it burns you up. Part of your being goes up in smoke. The black cinders of your flesh float away out there into space.

"I looked," he said. "I looked for the company but they were gone."

"A company man, Mr. Sherwin?"

He smiled gratefully. You *do* understand.

Were you a lonely kid, Mr. Sherwin? I can see you were a good boy. Good boys adopt companies later on. And companies adopt them. Cold parents, probably. Very orderly. Early toilet training.

He held up a yellow legal pad. He had written on every line. "Whereas the party of the first part, and the party of the second part, according to the agreement as contained herein, to heretofore acknowledge in fact, to said party in question . . ."

Harry wandered in. "This is Mr. Sherwin?" he asked. He shook his hand warmly.

"What do you have written there, on that pad, Mr. Sherwin?" Harry asked.

"Ipso and facto," Mr. Sherwin said.

"Really?"

"Yes. Ipso and facto. I wrote that. And whereas. That's there too. That is what all of those words say. It sums it up, wouldn't you say? The world situation? I made a pile out of words. I always liked words. Even as a child I got along well with words. I used them and they used me. I have stacked words. I have tasted words. Did you know that? I have tasted words, in my day."

"I can understand that, Mr. Sherwin," I said. "I personally think some words taste better than others."

Mr. Sherwin giggled. He liked that. He held his stomach tight with his arms. "I think so too. That's rich."

Harry smiled. We shared the urge to play word games with Mr. Sherwin.

"Listen," Mr. Sherwin said, "do you guys want me to read what it says here on this tablet? What it really says?"

We answered that we did.

"Well, it's a story. It's not really ipso facto. It's a real-life story in disguise. A secret story. Well, it's not a *secret* story. It's about this old guy . . ."

He began to read from the page that held the legalized nonsense. He read in a self-conscious, stilted way, the way a boy of eight or nine reads his composition in front of the class.

It was about an old man nobody knew. The old man had run away. Everything was too much for him. No one knew where the man had gone. But *he* knew where he was. He warned us to keep his secret.

"This old man does not know what to do with himself," he read. "No job. His daughter and son-in-law told him he was a bother. He got in their way. Crap, he knew that. What to do? What to do? No job. He plans on killing himself. He is so alone.

He doesn't know what to do with himself, see? If he kills himself, he will leave that hanging on his daughter. His daughter. Old Buddy herself. See, old Buddy used to ride with this old man, on the tractor on the farm. Old Buddy used to hop up on his lap. Doesn't Buddy love him anymore? Then, he figures, maybe it could be like it was once, long ago. Why not? Who says it can't be like it was?"

Mr. Sherwin paused. He turned to us. I smiled reassuringly. He went off, lost in his thoughts. We sat in silence for perhaps five minutes. Clearly he had gone away for now. We looked through his wallet. I found a telephone number. Harry dialed for the ambulance.

A woman answered my call.

"Yes?"

"I believe we have your father here at the clinic. I am Dr. Crain, a psychologist . . ."

"Oh, that's where he is." She spoke to someone in the background. "Do you know where that crazy man is, Ken? He is sitting in a psychologist's office. I'll bet he is sitting there telling you we don't care what happens to him. You know what his real problem is? He feels sorry for himself."

"We're going to send him to the hospital, lady. He's rather seriously disturbed right now."

"Oh," she said. She was quiet for a long time. I waited. "Can I talk to him?"

"If he can talk." He had momentarily taken his interest away from the world just like a little child who feels rejected and so he sulks and sucks his thumb.

He blinked himself awake. They talked. Mr. Sherwin's conversation was sane, even cheerful, at that moment. He and his daughter were meeting once more, but the meeting was brief and they parted. He seemed puzzled. Where was he? Where did he belong now? How do you hold on to a reality that is prying your fingers loose?

We watched as he slipped to the side of space, then down and away.

Furiously he began writing on the yellow-lined tablet. He

was a lonely child playing with words. He chose one. Grinned. He placed a word to his lips to taste. Mr. Sherwin will play like this until he grows tired of the game. Then he will sit his life away.

5

We are well into the new year. The winter sky is dark and overcast outside the big window overlooking Topanga Canyon Boulevard. It looks like rain. Harry draws the drapes and joins the small group gathered in the PET room telling sea stories. We compare notes and brag in subtle ways, one-upping one another. Harry moderates.

We share a quiet pride. Aren't we out in the forefront, where the action is? How many Beverly Hills analysts could handle this? What do theoreticians know about the real world? Do they know what it's like to deal with families screaming in pain or looking down at the floor in guilt for having one of their own dragged away by the psycho squad?

Harry answers the telephone. The caller on the other end must be a foreigner. "Yes," he says, "I understand . . . Repeat that? She burn the place down? She what . . . ?"

They talk on. We cannot follow the conversation from this end. Harry hangs up. "It's a goofy Chinese laundryman, Doc," he says. "He says we pick up his wife now. We take her to hospital. She crazy. She burn down laundry."

Inside the small Chinese laundry we saw two young men

working busily—one pressing clothes, the other tying and stacking bundles. They stopped working and stared at us, then continued on. An attractive Caucasian woman with copper-red hair, obviously dyed, was seated at a desk at the end of a long, narrow room that extended back to a partially screened apartment. She calmly rose and walked to the front desk where Harry and I were standing.

"She's in the back," she said. Her voice was strong and husky. A small, older Chinese man emerged from the rear apartment. He walked hurriedly toward us.

"She in there," he said, gesturing nervously. "She crazy. You take her away. You take her to nuthouse. She crazy lady. You take her now."

"Mister," I said, "we have to interview your wife before we even consider hospitalization."

"You take her! She crazy. She belong in nuthouse."

The red-head smiled. Her overconfidence was irritating. The young men—we deduced they were the man's sons—looked up, then returned to their work. The blonde went to get the woman, swinging her hips as she walked off. The two young men observed her impassively. Harry grimaced at me. What the hell was going on here?

The red-head beckoned to us from the rear of the shop. She shook her head, indicating the woman would not come out to talk to us. We walked back. An old stove and a single bed occupied the small rear room. The atmosphere in the room was dark and bleak. There was a heavy, undefinable smell, perhaps of spoiled vegetables.

A thin Chinese woman stood in the doorway. Her shabby pink dress was carelessly pinned together, revealing her thin brown legs and knobby knees. The small front pockets were stuffed full of odds and ends—paper, bits of cloth. She faced us. Her eyes were absolutely petrified.

The red-head approached her. She shrank back. "Come on, dear," the woman said sweetly. "These men want to talk to you."

"Argh!" she screamed. "Argh. Gawh!" She clutched herself protectively. She ran, huddling in the corner of the room.

"Dear," the woman said, "please take it easy. No one is going to hurt you."

"Let me try to talk to her," I said.

The Chinese man stuck his head in. "She crazy! She burn up store." He jumped around, imitating flames licking at the walls of his laundry. "You take her away now."

"What George is saying," the woman said patronizingly, "is that Mrs. Song has been cooking her own meals on this stove. Sometimes the poor thing forgets to turn it off. She has ruined several pans. She almost burned up the place last week."

"Why is she doing her own cooking?"

"Oh, we don't live here. Nobody lives here. Well, she does. We live in Los Angeles. That's part of the difficulty. No one here to supervise her. I'm the housekeeper for the boys. I keep the books. Mr. Song hired me to help the boys with their English."

I turned to the Chinese woman. "Could you sit down?" I asked her.

"No! No!" She shrieked. "Kill me! Kill me! Argh!"

I reluctantly told Harry we had better call the ambulance. He nodded sadly. She was completely helpless. Undernourished. And she *could* burn the place down.

The boys stood in the doorway. "Who want laundry done in crazy place?" Mr. Song shouted. "Crazy lady scream! Burn down store!" The boys looked at their mother without emotion.

The Chinese lady walked to the middle of the room. She raised her arms over her head like a bullfighter ready to stick the bull. Her fingers were spread wide apart. She jumped around in some wild, mad ritual, throwing her long black hair over her shoulder. She stopped and stared at me. Her eyes were frightening in their intensity. I felt that I must not look into her eyes for long. Something terrible would happen to me. She began wiggling her fingers like crawling snakes. Was she hexing me?

She jabbered away, some loud, sing-song incantation in

Chinese. She dropped her head down. Her long black hair rolled around in the air, covering her face. She grabbed some empty space in her hands, raised it up to show me, and threw it at me. She smiled mockingly. She pointed a long, thin, accusative finger in the face of the caucasian woman. She looked at me inquiringly, momentarily lucid. Did I see the situation here?

"She fuck. She fuck! She fuck everybody! Sons!" she screamed.

Inadvertently I said, "No." I caught her eyes. She was gone now. Withdrawn inside.

The red-head's calm indifference diminished, the effects of the mad ritual. She looked away disdainfully.

The Chinese lady was not done. She began another dance to show us what had been done to her. She aged before our eyes. She was dead now. A mechanical thing. She collapsed on the small bed.

Quietly we sat together, the six of us, waiting for the ambulance. An hour passed. Harry and I paced, cursing the ambulance company. The woman lay quietly on the bed staring into space, frozen in some inner terror. The boys glanced at her, then looked away. Harry walked outside, finally saying, "Here they come, Doc."

Two men and a woman rushed into the quiet of the room. "Grab her, Doc," Harry said. He reached for her shoulders. I grabbed her legs. She weighed almost nothing. She was trembling like a frightened little bird.

"Honey," the woman attendant said, leaning over her, "nobody is going to hurt you."

She stroked her cheek gently. Harry strapped her wrists together, tying her to the gurney. I removed the contents of her pockets. Old pieces of cloth, bits of paper, match folders, buttons. Her earthly possessions. Little signposts pointing nowhere.

From a distance we heard the wail of a scream that began somewhere back in the woman's chest. It got louder and louder, more insistent, more urgent. It hit the room like some flat metal object. It was her final scream for help, her scream of rage. A wild, primitive scream, it echoed its finality against unseen deep canyons and thick granite walls, emerging from time past into the present. The lady was screaming for her unlived life.

6

It has been oddly quiet for a PET day. Not a single telephone call or walk-in. Harry busies himself with his PET records.

Al Johnson enters the office. "Quiet day?" he asks.

"Shouldn't I get as much money as the police?" Harry complains. "Look at all my responsibilities."

"PET can be a bitch," Al says. "I don't like PET much. These people are really crazy."

It's the game players that bug him, Al says. People who think that life is some kind of game.

"They're a pain in the ass," Al muses. "Once this old guy called the clinic. He said he was definitely going to kill himself, and right away. So if we didn't want him to die, see, we had better get right over there. However, he *might* wait, he said. He just might, but he wasn't sure. Well, I *knew* he was conning me, but I also knew this is how some suicides work. So right away I called the fire rescue squad. 'Look,' I said, 'there is this old guy, and he says he . . .' Then I stopped because I realized I hadn't gotten his address."

He looks at Harry, then at me. We shrug. No reason to be

embarrassed. It could happen to anyone. "So I sat around, naturally, figuring the old guy was busying himself with the mechanics of his suicide, and I had really blown it. Fortunately he called back. He sounded disappointed. 'You didn't get my address,' he said, like I had rejected him.

"The psychiatrist and I arrived at this raunchy old hotel on Ventura Boulevard," Al says. "We knocked. Got no answer, so we walked in. The TV was blaring. The room was empty. My stomach dropped down into my shoes. The old man was probably in the bathroom bleeding to death, or hanging from the shower bar. Neither of us wanted to lead the way. Finally I got the nerve to peek in. The shower curtain was drawn. You should have seen Dr. Brown. Jesus, his face was white. I was rapidly getting nauseous. I managed to pull the curtain back . . ."

Al pauses. He is playing it for the suspense.

"What? What happened?" We respond in a high-pitched chorus.

"Nothing, naturally. It was empty. The shower was empty."

"So?"

"Nothing."

"So where was the old guy?"

"Well, the old prick came sauntering in from the outside about a minute later. He was all gleeful and pleased with himself, though he pretended he didn't know what the fuss was all about.

"That's nuts!" Harry says. "Nuts!"

Why would someone want to play a trick like that? Harry says it is a bid for attention. The old man felt very powerful controlling the situation like that, getting the big red rescue truck out, just for him. We could observe omnipotence at first hand.

This old guy probably had nobody in the world who cared about him. Still, there was a game involved. He was playing with life.

Harry says he could do without some of these acts. This

old man specifically should shape up his act. Would he actually kill himself someday soon? We look at one another. Our gazes are neutral, businesslike. Harry returns to his papers and mumbles. "Fuck! I ought to get more money!"

*   *

A cold rain falls outside. It has been a wet February. It is eerie, I think, this idea of different worlds. Here we are on the second floor of this new, carpeted office building. Another world goes about its silent business outside. We cannot hear the rain on the windows or the steps of the miniature people below. The cars crawl quietly along the wet streets, and it all seems unreal. One world out there. Another world in here. And then the private, designing world of an old guy with a really terrible sense of humor.

7

The young attorney with the smooth skin and soft blue eyes introduced himself as Lance Goldenrod's lawyer. He stood beside the receptionist's desk with the easy self-confidence of the fraternity man who seriously wonders why other people are dumb enough to be born dark or poor.

"Lance Goldenrod?" I asked, trying not to smile at the name.

It irritated him and threw him off that I hadn't heard of

him. He shifted his feet. "He's a rock star, Doctor," he said patiently. "He's made several films."

I turned to Harry. "Have you ever heard of Lance Goldenrod?" He said he hadn't.

"He's been getting bugged by this young woman who claims she's his wife," the lawyer said quietly. "She is obviously psychotic."

"We don't know that," Harry said.

"I believe you will agree with me when you look over this material." He handed me a large manila envelope.

He examined the plastic nameplate on my desk, brushing some dust away, then absently examined his fingertips. "You're a psychologist?"

I nodded. I began running over the material he had given me. There were several long, rambling love letters to Lance, written in a childlike scrawl, and a telegram. Other letters were addressed to his manager and attorney.

"She says here that Lance's law firm is a bunch of pussies and fags," I said. "Obviously the young woman is delusional."

"She exaggerates," he said mildly.

I began reading aloud for Harry's benefit. "As you are well aware and entirely cognitive of, I am and continue to be the sole and legal wife of Lance Goldenrod. Self-said Lance continues to ignore said facts and consequently denies my existence and status as his legal, sole, and faithful wife. He has been further aided and abetted by his so-called and alleged attorneys, who constitute a group of types best and accurately described as pussies and fags, each and every one of said attorneys . . ."

The tone shifted. It appealed to Lance to acknowledge to others and to his adoring public that she was indeed his legal and faithful wife. Why did he insist on denying that he knew her so very well and personally? Why did he avoid her eyes when he passed her in the hallway at the television studio and pretend he did not hear her shouts at him to pay attention to her? Please, she pleaded, pay attention. Then she added the angry, desperate words that denounced that "bitch with the big tits who stands in the way of our earthly and spiritual happiness claiming she is the rightful and legal Mrs. Lance Goldenrod."

"If this imposter does not stand aside," she continued, "I will be forced to take any and all necessary actions, none of which are to be stated openly at this time."

"That's a threat on his life," the lawyer said. His soft blue eyes were icy cold. His checked cashmere sport coat must have cost him two hundred dollars.

"I'm not sure . . ." I said.

"Doctor, we can take this young woman to court; that's no problem. I can have her arrested in half an hour. We are only trying to handle it all without a big fuss. And what about the young woman?"

My face reddened. They had it all figured out. They knew we would want to avoid a messy arrest of an emotionally disturbed young woman. If we committed her then Lance was home free. She was a groupie, most likely, and he had taken advantage of the situation. I told the attorney we would make a home visit.

As we drove along, Harry recalled seeing the rock star on television. He was a slight little guy with a cute mustache and a weak voice. The teenyboppers were crazy about him. One of Harry's daughters loved him dearly. Harry hadn't wanted to give the attorney the satisfaction of admitting he had heard of him.

"They want to mother the mother," Harry said. "I should think they would be more discriminating. Son of a bitch is a . . ."

"I know," I said. "A bony-assed white man."

"Right on *time,*" he said. "You're getting the idea. My daughter argues with me when I put these wimps down, Doc. She tells me white people are human beings. What do you think?"

We drove along an unimproved road that wound through an older and poorer section of the valley, past small commercial establishments, Mexican cafés, Volkswagen repair shops. Several bars advertised topless entertainment and cowboy music on Friday and Saturday nights, dancing girls with lunch.

"I used to hang around this neck of the woods years back," Harry said. "Three years ago this was all onions."

We stopped at the manager's office of the apartment building. The grizzly old manager checked our IDs carefully. He looked at Harry, then down at his card, then up again. Harry shuffled irritably. The manager was small, pudgy, and grimy.

"So what do you want with her?" he asked.

"I told you," I said. "We have a complaint and we want to ask her a few questions."

"I don't understand," he said.

"We won't go inside unless she lets us in," I said.

It was Harry, evidently. The manager simply could not accept the authority of a black man.

A tall, exceptionally pretty girl with long auburn hair opened the door just as I placed my finger on the bell. There was no trace of emotional disturbance. Her smile was wide and friendly. She threw her hair to the side in that practiced gesture of the attractive girl calling attention to herself.

"Hello," she said warmly. "What can I do for you gentlemen?"

"We would like to talk to you for a few minutes."

"Sure, come on in."

We had not introduced ourselves. I wanted to tell her that she should not welcome two men into her apartment like this. Could we have the wrong apartment? Maybe she had gotten herself miraculously cured.

We surveyed the front room. It was clean and fresh. There were cut flowers on the coffee table in front of the sofa where we were seated. An ironing board in the middle of the room was stacked high with ironing.

"We are from the Department of Mental Health," I said finally.

"I know," she said. "I knew you were coming. Lance sent you, didn't he?"

"Not exactly."

"His attorney, right?" She wasn't upset enough. She smiled reflectively. "Well, I knew you would be here today. They refuse to accept the facts, that's all."

She picked up the iron. She ran it lightly over a well-worn white blouse. As she ironed she hummed softly, ignoring our presence. She had forgotten us. Harry pointed to the floor. *The cord wasn't plugged in.*

"You gentlemen think I'm insane, don't you?"

"No," Harry said impulsively. "Of course not. We are just here to make an evaluation . . ."

"You have children, don't you? I can tell."

"Yes."

"How many?"

"Two," Harry said.

"That's what I thought. I have certain powers, you know. I can tell you're a very sensitive man." She smiled warmly. "Attractive too."

"Well, thank you," Harry said. "You're very attractive. Isn't she, Doc?"

"I'll say."

"I have good hair," she said. "It is my best feature. Lance said my long auburn hair was my best feature. You know Lance?"

"Not exactly. We've heard of him, though."

"I'm psychic," she said. "Sometimes I can read people's thoughts. I knew you were coming today. I *am* his wife, you know." She grimaced. "Lance doesn't deny it. He talked to me last night."

"Really?"

She laughed lightly. "Oh, I know you don't believe me. I can tell. I'm afraid you're just like the others."

"Well, that telegram you sent him . . ." I said.

She stared at me. Her eyes seemed cold suddenly. "I was angry," she said. "He was denying we were man and wife. And I saw him with that ugly bitch with the big tits who claims she's his wife."

"You said some pretty terrible things. Actually his lawyers could prosecute you for threatening his life, you know. That's why we are here. We have to check you out . . ."

"Oh, I knew they would deny it." She was calm again. "I knew they would say I was insane."

She began ironing rapidly. I thought her legs were too strong for her to be too disturbed. Harry glanced at me. What to do? She was out of it, obviously. But we couldn't just talk her into hospitalization. And she wouldn't get any help on her own.

"Lance hasn't been too good to me lately," she said idly. "He denies that we are man and wife. Poor Lance. Of course it's that bitch! She has her claws in him." She smiled at me warmly. "He's so sweet. That bitch is killing him! That bitch is eating him alive."

She turned, facing me. "She will get hers." Her eyes narrowed into a hard, frightening stare. Harry looked down. She seemed to be considering some terrible, murderous plan. Her face had transformed before our eyes. Something evil and dark now possessed her. She grinned at me lewdly. She ran her tongue over her lips. Jesus, I thought, this pretty young thing is a cannibal.

Harry fixed his eyes on the iron in her hand. She could decide to throw it. I was her enemy now and I didn't know how to extricate myself. The fragile girl reclaimed her body. She smiled at me kindly and began humming to herself.

"Don't you think Lance is the best?" That dark look again.

"Well, he's popular," Harry said. "I'll say that."

"Goddamn mother fucker! Son of a bitch!" She switched off, becoming gentle. "I *am* Mrs. Lance Goldenrod."

It was too much. Harry looked around for the telephone. "Where the hell is the phone? Do you have a phone?" he asked. "I want to call the office. I forgot to tell my secretary where we were going."

"Yes, there is the telephone."

"Where is it?"

"In the bedroom."

He returned. "It's dead."

"Yes, they shut off my service. They said I was without sufficient funds. Why would they say that?"

Harry excused himself and headed downstairs to the manager's office. She continued her ironing. She turned her back to me. She was aware of me in a new way. I could not see her face, but I was sure that the witchlike possession had taken over once more. Her back was stiff. My heart pounded. I prepared to duck.

She turned, facing me. It was the soft, distracted pretty girl again. "Let me show you something," she said. I sat. "Oh, come on," she said. "I won't eat you up, silly." She walked toward the back of the apartment. Her hips swayed; Follow me, they said. I remained seated. My emotions were mixed. Attraction and repulsion. Fear and protectiveness. It was making me anxious. Where was Harry?

She stood there with her hands on her hips. She smiled at me challengingly. She gestured with her head. Come on, she said, join me.

"Look," I said, "we have to do this evaluation of you and . . ."

She turned and picked up a bulky picture frame. She sat down on the couch next to me. Her thigh brushed mine. She stared into my face inquiringly. I looked away.

She opened the picture frame. I saw two eight-by-ten glossy photos. One was an obvious publicity photo of Lance. The other was a photograph of herself. They seemed to be smiling at each other. The effect was that of two young people who seemed to belong together. Lance does know this girl, I thought. Maybe they were married. Or maybe he had promised to marry her and then she had become more obviously disturbed.

I heard footsteps. The ambulance had arrived.

She ran to the window. "What are you doing? What are you *doing!*"

Harry ran in. He grabbed her arms. The ambulance attendants entered.

She stared hard into my eyes. "Do you know what you're doing?" she screamed. "Do you know what you're doing?"

8

A middle-aged ex-military policeman walked into the clinic. Though he now worked in an auto parts plant, he still held himself proudly and rigidly as he described his early life with a mother who had gradually gone mad. His father had left several years earlier. Now his mother was his responsibility.

"That's a lot to carry," I said.

"I know." He looked down at the floor. He had asked for help before, but it still embarrassed him. He looked up. "She can't help herself," he said. "She tries. She really tries."

His mother disappeared for months at a time. Or she was placed in a hospital. She had been hospitalized a number of times. And somehow she always pulled herself together and got released quickly.

"My mother is a very courageous woman," he said, more with sadness than with pride.

"That's a big load you are carrying," Harry said. "Maybe you ought to just . . ."

"I know. But I can't leave her on her own. Not when she calls for help. Sometimes she . . . sometimes she . . . she gets all involved with . . . with old winos."

The young man began to sob. Then he cried openly, the way a little kid cries, his face breaking apart. He rubbed his eyes with his fists and said, "Well, let's go get her again, OK? Please don't let her talk you into thinking she's sane. Please. She is very clever. And she absolutely *despises* the state hospitals. They scare her to death."

The thin, fragile woman we saw standing in the distance appeared lost, terribly lost. I first spotted her behind the Westval Market standing frozen in the warm February sun, and I could see and feel at a hundred yards that this human being was without anchorage, without footing.

"You go talk to her, Doc," Harry said. "I'll wait back here by the car. Where's her son? He said he would follow us here."

I walked toward her. I could sense her panic. She felt every step of my advance. Were her shoulders shaking? She raised her chin in a gesture of panicky defiance. That is rare courage, I thought. It made me aware of my steps, the sound of my shoes on the pavement. I could see myself through her eyes, the insistent approach of this dark stranger. My feet sounded flat and meaningless on the asphalt. Plop, plop, plop.

I was three feet from her now. Her face was so pretty, so ravaged. She was surprisingly tall. Very thin, a skeleton almost. Her features were sharp. Her eyes were ringed with the shadows of the darkness she lived in. The demons had been at work inside her doing their typical violence. She stared at me and I had the idea that she could see right through me, right into my innards.

Her son had arrived. Good! He parked his little VW next to the big, gray county wagon. He emerged slowly. He had been through this before. He seemed so tired. He began his long, slow walk across the black asphalt to greet his insane mother.

She was shaking all over. "What do you *want?*" she screamed. She knew why we were there.

"I'm from the County Department of Mental Health, ma'm," I said. I showed her my identification. She didn't read it. The picture on the front looked like a Mafia chief smiling. She held my wallet in her trembling hand. "What does that have to do with me? A card?"

"It gives me the right to . . ."

"Who says? *Who says!*" Passers-by, off in the distance, paused to consider the problem. Was he raping this woman?

I walked over to the car. The doors were wide open. I saw milk cartons, letters strewn about, a sad old sweater. There were loaves of unwrapped bread, a faded blanket, and a large sack of potatoes. The interior of the automobile reflected her inner confusion and chaos. Fresh food, yet she appeared to be starving. The cover of the driver's seat had a gaping hole in the wrong place, toward the front. I pictured her hunched forward, her nose near the windshield, driving madly into some future.

"Why did you bring these men here?" She raised her arms threateningly, extending her fingers.

"I had to, Mother. Jesus, you need help. You aren't eating, for one thing. Jesus." Her son's eyes welled with tears.

"You invoke the Lord?" she screamed. "You invoke the Lord! You people are the ones who need help. Is it against the law to live in a car? Is it? Answer me! *Is it?*"

She pushed her face into her son's. "Do I know you?"

He recoiled, dropping his head down. "Mama . . ." he said.

He looked ashamed and exposed. He stood stiffly at attention. He was being a good boy, a good soldier. How many times had he experienced this drama? How many times had he watched her as she abandoned him, leaving him alone in this world as she entered another? He turned to me. "Can't you see that she is . . ."

"I'm not your mother." She grinned shrewdly. "I'm nobody's mother." She glanced quickly at me. Almost slipped there. She stiffened. "I'm no mother to someone who would bring people from the Department of . . . whatever, asking stupid questions. People who have problems of their own."

The M.P. looked at me. "What kind of evidence you need? Get her to tell you about the demons."

"We have to have definite evidence that she is not in contact. She hasn't said anything . . ."

"Ask her why she leaves the car doors open," the M.P. said resignedly.

"All right. Why, lady? Why do you leave the car doors open?"

She smirked. "Tell me this. Is there any law against leaving car doors open? Is there? Have you ever read a law that says human beings cannot, now or in the future, leave their car doors open, in the interest of ventilation?"

She turned to her son. "*You,*" she said, hate in her voice.

He broke into tears. "Fuck!" he yelled. "Ask her about the doors. Ask her!"

"That's enough," I said. I decided to push her, to have something definite to write down on the application.

"Lady," I said, "tell me the truth about those doors. I want the truth."

"The truth?" She was shaken. She knew I was going to push at those tenuous defenses of hers. "I leave those doors open," she said haltingly, "to air out the car. Anybody knows that."

"I'm sorry," I said. "Explain that, will you? I don't understand."

"To air out the car! To air out the Chevy. The *car.* To air it out!" She was getting agitated.

"What's wrong with the windows?"

"Nothing is wrong with the windows." She grinned. "Well," she said, "that does it."

"What do you mean?"

"Anybody knows that." She shuffled her feet. Then, still grinning, she left the scene. Like the Cheshire cat, she left no more than a smile to remember her by. "They are too big for those little windows," she said softly, more to herself. "They would complain about that. They don't like to crawl out of little windows."

I signaled for Harry. I wondered sadly at this goofy need for evidence, this searching of the personal premises with so dubious a warrant.

9

"Get on the extension there, Doc," Harry said.

I pushed the extension button. "This is Dr. Crain," Harry said, "I want him to listen in. Now, would you tell him what you just told me?"

"It's my husband." She sounded black. "It's . . . he is mentally ill. I know that's what is bothering him. He says . . . I am possessed, you know?"

"Possessed?"

"By the devil. He says the devil is making me flirt with other men and is sending out messages to them, telling them I want to . . . you know, have intercourse with them, and it's the devil who makes me wiggle when I walk." She sobbed. "I can't help it, how I walk. I just walk . . ."

We told her we would make a home visit. Were there any weapons? No. Yes! He had a gun somewhere. He brought it home from the service. He never used it. Would she please try to find it and hide it somewhere? Yes. Was he a big man? Pretty big. How big was pretty big? Six-foot two. He weighed two hundred pounds and he lifted weights.

"We'll be right over," I said, swallowing. "It could be a little messy."

She understood. We hung up. I realized I was tense when I heard myself talking loudly, running over the details. Harry called the police. He explained the situation. Two cars—four men.

"I am going to get those mothers to lead the way in, Doc, if it kills . . ."

"Right," I said.

Their home was fifteen minutes away, toward the low hills to the south, in an older section of the valley.

This young man could be dangerous. He might want to kill the devil—and he might have to shoot his wife to get at him.

Harry licked his dry lips and began to whistle. We drove in silence. As we approached the general area we saw a helicopter circling a shopping center. As we got closer we could see red lights flashing all about. Ten squad cars were parked along the narrow street. Policemen were milling all about.

"Someone," Harry said, "has his wires crossed. We only requested two cars."

A tall policeman approached the county car. "Are you the men from the psycho unit?" His voice was flat and unemotional. "We understand there's a madman running around loose here—a real psycho. He's armed and dangerous. Is that right?"

"Look," I said. "We didn't want all of this . . ." I looked toward the house. What was the man doing right at this moment? What was he thinking about all this commotion? Did she get the gun? Did he have it pointed at us right now? At *me?*

"An escapee from Cam, right?" The officer spoke like an actor portraying a policeman.

"No, not exactly. Look," Harry said, "we don't need all of this hardware here. We only wanted . . ."

The helicopter swooped down noisily. It stopped in midair thirty feet above our heads. Harry looked up nervously.

"I hate them fuckers," he said angrily. He turned to the policeman. "Your sergeant has got the message all fucked up.

I mean this is a fuckup. We only asked for two cars." He slammed the car door. We stood together, helpless and bewildered.

The policeman spoke again from deep within his throat. "We understand there is a madman, a real psycho, loose in that house over there. He is armed and dangerous. Is that right?"

Policemen began positioning themselves strategically. Guns were trained on the house. A lieutenant in civilian clothes approached, carrying a bull horn.

"Harry," I said, "this is out of hand, completely out of hand. What'll we do?"

What could we do? We couldn't leave. It was our esponsibility to *protect* the man now. *What if they decided to open fire* for Christ's sake?

Harry shuffled his feet. He looked at me anxiously He glanced upward at the helicopter. It scooted off suddenly, then backed into a circular run, its propellers whirling in a frant'c whine. "Do we need *that?*" Harry asked.

"You never know," the cop said. "You never know. We heard there was a madman . . ."

"Well, won't the guy be forewarned?" I shouted. "Won't he suspect something?"

Harry glanced at me. "Some sense of humor you got," he said.

A short, pudgy, black woman approached us. She was distraught. She wiped her hands on the side of her skirt. "What's happening? Are you the gentlemen I talked to? What *is* all this?"

I shrugged. "Lady, we didn't . . . Look, where is your husband?"

"Doc," Harry said, "we are not going into that house. No way. That guy probably has a bead on us right at this moment. I'll bet he has that gun pointed . . ."

"No," she said. "Please."

"I'll bet that son of a bitch is aiming his gun right at us at this moment, Doc. I'll bet."

"No," she said.

"Let's call the whole damned thing off, Doc," he said. "Let's go on back to the clinic and start over. What do you think?"

"No," she said.

"How are you going to do it, Harry? All of those cops. What if they won't listen to us?"

"You wait here." He walked over to the lieutenant with the bull horn. They talked. They began arguing. The officer was angry. He was refusing to leave. Harry pulled out his ID. The officer read it carefully. Harry was showing him we had the authority. Finally the man nodded. He would gather in the troops.

Harry returned. "Did it, Doc," he said smugly. "Did it."

"No," the young woman said. "Don't leave. He's sick. He really is. You don't have to be afraid of him. He's asleep, I think. Anyway, I hid the gun."

"You *hid* the gun?" I said. "Boy."

The helicopter slid away in the air. It flew sideways into the smog over the foothills. The cars began driving off.

Frantically Harry signaled to the lieutenant. He ignored him. The ambulance had arrived. Harry told the attendants to wait.

A thin young man appeared on the porch of the house. He was una ed and looked perplexed. He rubbed his eyes in the sun. Ha ry g anced at the young woman. Yes, this was her husband. We walked over.

"What he hell is going on?" he asked. "What's all the commotion? I could have sworn I heard a helicopter right over the top o he house. What's happening?" He stared at the three of us suspiciou ly.

' I don't know," I said. "Something was happening. I don't know exactly what it was all about."

"What did all those cops want? What was going on?"

Hi wife looked down.

Ha d to tell," Harry said. "Say, do you suppose we could talk to you for a few minutes?"

"What about?"

"It's county business."

"County business?" He shrugged. "All right. Come on in."

We followed him in. "You fellows want a cup of coffee?" he asked. He glanced at his wife. She smoothed her skirt self-consciously.

We sat down on the couch. The wife sank deep into an upholstered chair opposite. I hadn't realized how small she was. She looked like a frightened little girl. She stared at us as if she wanted to tell us something urgent but could not think of the words.

He brought in cups of coffee on a tray. He sat on the arm of his wife's chair. "So what will we talk about?"

I was embarrassed. "Well, we just wanted to discuss things. You know . . ."

"Like what?"

I looked at Harry for help. He grinned. "Oh, things."

"Are you embarrassed? I used to get embarrassed. That was before I found Christ."

"You found Christ?"

"Yes."

His wife sighed heavily. She rose and walked toward the kitchen. She really did wiggle rather seductively. Her husband watched her until she left the room. He turned to me inquiringly, as if to ask me if I had observed her walk. Did I see what he saw?

"My wife is a very attractive woman," he said ominously. "Don't you think?"

"Well, yes, she is," I said. "She definitely is."

He turned to Harry. "What do you think? Do you agree?"

"Oh, yeah," Harry said. "Sure."

"She is possessed by the devil. You see, it is the devil that makes you look at her when she walks. And the devil makes her walk like that. The devil makes men look at her desirous of carnal relations."

Harry walked to the front door. He signaled to the ambulance attendants. They approached the house warily.

"Come on in," Harry said. "It's all right."

The two men in white stood in the doorway.

"Who are you?" the young man asked. "What do you want?"

They did not answer. "We think maybe you had better go to the hospital," I said.

"What for?" he shouted. "I'm not sick."

"Well, we think you need a short stay in the hospital. Maybe just a couple of days. They'll give you some medication. It will help you, so you won't see things, you know. About the devil and all that."

He bolted. We grabbed him. Harry twisted his arm behind his back. He screamed. We subdued him quickly, strapping him to the gurney.

"The devil!" he screamed as they rolled the gurney to the ambulance parked up the street. "She is possessed by the devil. He is making you do this to me!"

The ambulance drove off. We talked to the young woman for a few minutes. She sighed, finally. She was very tired, she said. She wanted to go to bed. She rubbed her stomach gently, suggestively. She smiled at us. She turned and walked into the house, her ass wiggling as if it had a mind of its own.

10

The telephone was buzzing just as we returned to the clinic. An apartment manager was calling about one of his tenants creating a disturbance.

The tenant was a pleasant woman in her early fifties. Her face was mottled from heavy drinking. Books and magazines were scattered about. Laundry was piled high on the couch.

"Look at these legs," the woman said. "God, my skin is so white it's ridiculous. And my arms. Look how skinny I am. I'm a mess. And as a housekeeper I'm worse than Phyllis Diller. You should see my kitchen. It's filthy."

"You dig at yourself a lot, don't you?" Harry said.

"Well, it's true. I'm a mess. Look at this place. It's a disgrace."

"Sure," I said.

"Really, I am. It's true."

"Do you ever say positive things about yourself?"

"There isn't anything good about me." She laughed. It was a kind of burst, a small explosion. It seemed to please her, talking negatively this way.

"You read a lot," I said.

"Yeah, I like to keep up. It's about all I do, really. Most of the time I just hide under the covers. I'm a coward. I'm really lazy. I don't do anything except hide or drink wine. What did you say you fellows wanted?"

"The manager here thought we ought to look in on you," Harry said kindly. "He thinks maybe you are . . . you know, too lonely." He paused. He did not know how to continue.

I picked it up. "He said you create a fuss sometimes . . ."

"A fuss?"

"You know, a disturbance. Bothering other tenants."

"Well, it's possible. Maybe I bother them when I dump my wine bottles into the metal trash can. Do I play my radio too loud? I probably do. I am absolutely oblivious to other people's needs most of the time. I'm very selfish. All I think about is . . ."

"It's more than that," Harry said. "But look, we don't see you as mentally disturbed, or in danger to yourself or to others . . ."

"I'm a drunk," she said. "I've been drinking heavily for two years now. Not that I didn't drink before."

"Something happen?" Harry asked.

"My husband left, left me for a young woman. I deserved it, the way I treated him. I don't blame him. Who would want to . . . you know, with this . . . ?"

She stretched her thin legs out. They really weren't much. She had varicose veins and blotchy skin. "I look like a plucked chicken. What do you think?"

"Oh, no," Harry said. "I wouldn't say that."

She did look like a plucked chicken.

She smiled in the certainty of her thousand obvious deficiencies. "I don't blame him. Who would want to be married to a drunk like me?"

"But you weren't a drunk before."

"I was selfish."

"You take everything out on yourself."

We talked awhile. She gave us coffee. She was an intelligent woman. Very well read. At one point she mentioned that they had been married for twenty-six years. What really hurt her feelings, she said, was the way he told her. He said he hadn't loved her in maybe ten years. So what was she supposed to do with *her* memory of those ten years?

Another thing that bothered her was the little Mexican—the young woman who stole him from her. ("It was obviously my fault.") When did he meet her? What bothered her was she had not even sensed what was going on. It meant she hadn't been sensitive to his feelings at all. This was proof she was a lousy wife. Selfish.

"You live here all by yourself," I said. "You must get pretty lonely."

"I do get lonely," she said. "I stay in bed a lot. I hide under the covers."

"Well, you just had quite a blow to your pride," I said. "To say the least."

"I'm just lazy," she said with conviction.

"You shouldn't pick on yourself so much. It's not good for you," I said.

"It's all true."

She looked up at me. She was agonized, terribly afraid. Please, she seemed to say, please let me berate myself. Don't you see that I must? I'll dissolve, I'll disappear, I'll be lost if I give in to my sorrow. This way I am in some control.

"Well," I said lamely, "you don't have many people to talk to. Maybe that's why you're bothering the neighbors at night."

She laughed a curious sneeze-laugh, spraying the air around her. "You find things to talk to, living alone. I talk to bugs. Naturally I talk to myself."

A small spider walked across the newspaper on the floor in front of us as if on cue. "Like him, see. I'll talk to him. Hi, little bug. Hi there. Like that. Crazy, right?"

Harry was curious about her conversation with the little spider. "No," he said earnestly, "that's not crazy. I sometimes talk to my plants."

"I do that," she said. "And my bird."

She buried her head in her hands. Harry walked over and put his hand on her shoulder.

"It's the memories," she said. "How do I remember everything different—like it wasn't the way I remember it?"

"Last week I decided that when he came over to give me

my check I wasn't going to talk to him about anything but business matters. Then when he walked in the door I started babbling like a . . ." She covered her face with her hands, sobbing heavily.

Harry massaged her shoulder lightly, impulsively, in a quick, desperate motion. She placed her hand over his. This woman had not had much physical contact lately.

We left soon afterward. I asked her to call me the following Monday. Maybe I should have warned her firmly that she had better get control of herself. She had no awareness of pounding on the walls in the middle of the night and of screaming obscenities about young Mexican whores and men who fuck everything in sight and leave you so alone, so *alone,* at fifty-five.

Harry said that the Lanterman-Petris-Short Act didn't say so specifically, but the way he read it you had to be crazy around the clock, and she was only crazy in the middle of the night, so she didn't qualify.

* *

"This has been a rough day, Doc," Harry said. "Three calls is two calls too many in a single afternoon. One in the morning and one in the afternoon is plenty."

We drove back slowly through the rural area of Tarzana. We passed the Motion Picture Home and Hospital where some of the old actors and actresses were housed until they died.

We spoke of relationships, how people expected too much of others. All this talk of "shoulds," all these rational new rules angered me. "You should be over him by now." People putting time limits on feelings. The lady who talked to her bugs bothered me more than most.

I mentioned a man I had seen at a clinic years back. Old George Randall. His wife died suddenly. They had been very close. He brought her coffee in bed on Saturday mornings, and one morning when he brought in the coffee she was dead. So he took off all his clothes—they lived on the second story of an apartment building—and he screamed his anguish to the world.

Naturally they locked old George up in the psychiatric ward. He wasn't ready to give up his wife. Not by a long shot. She wasn't gone yet, he said. He could feel her all around him. He took himself over to a corner of the dayroom so he could get away from all the noise and talk with her better. He had so much left he hadn't said.

A young psychiatrist asked him why he was refusing to socialize with the other patients. He "shouldn't" be here off by himself, he said. He "should" accept his wife's death. Maybe they would have to give him shock treatments if he was disoriented in time and space. George was too stubborn to tell the young man what month it was. He told me later that he knew perfectly well what month it was. He wasn't sure about the day, though.

The point was George Randall wasn't crazy. It was the *expectations* that were crazy.

Harry ignored my tirade. He drove along, whistling softly. "I'm a sex fiend," he said. "Do you always know what day it is, Doc? I never know. And if you asked me those mental status questions, to tell the truth, I'd fail."

He lit up a small cigar confidently. "I can never remember what day it is. Only Fridays and payday. That's it. And Sunday, sometimes."

11

It was a cold, windy day in early March. Sitting in the PET car, I watched the big red and white ambulance roll off down the quiet valley street. I was eating a tuna fish sandwich and wondering about the different personalities that houses have. Not people—houses. We had just sent a nice middle-aged lady off to Camarillo and were still suffering from the minor shock of realizing the goings-on in that particular house perched drunkenly on its lot.

It was a madhouse. When we opened its front door we entered some inner sanctum. We felt the eerie chill of the place, Harry and I. The air seemed thinner in that dark, lonely living room. It was a house without a soul. Which meant the woman whose home it once was had lost *her* soul. Aren't women's houses a direct reflection of the state of their being? Surely every therapist knows where his woman client is, psychologically, by the way she describes her home. "My house is a mess," she says. She feels messy inside. "I'm fixing up my house," she says excitedly. She is feeling positive, more confident, pleased with her inner self.

The house I was looking at was definitely mad. It exuded insanity. Its window eyes and its door made an unfunny face, dead as a Halloween pumpkin. One eye was closed permanently, as if struck by a heavy blow. The other empty eye, ignoring such adversity, winked inappropriately.

"Harry," I asked, a bit reluctantly, "do you think houses can be crazy just like people?"

Harry mused on the question. "Of course I do, Doc. You know I do. As a matter of fact, I give that a lot of thought—how houses can go crazy just like people. I give that a *lot* of thought." He raised his eyes to a psychiatrist in the sky. "And cars, Doc. Cars have their problems . . ."

"I'm serious," I said. "Look at that house. Look at it. Now isn't that a crazy house?"

He studied it. "As a matter of fact, it is. Let's you and me seventy-two that mother house, Doc."

We laughed, but our hearts weren't in it. There were so many questions that would never be answered. A teenager had called the office regarding her mother, who, she said—too blandly, I thought—had flipped. From the description she gave, the mother had lost contact with reality. She was hearing voices, talking to herself. Worse yet, that morning she had chased a neighbor down the street, wielding a long two-by-four with a big nail in the end of it.

We were met by the daughter. She was a small, very dark-skinned girl who greeted us with a sly smile. She wore skin-tight shorts and a loose-fitting, revealing blouse. Her small breasts jiggled as she led us into the cold, dark, barren living room. She looked down at her breasts and then up again, indicating her wish that we soak in her charms. When my eyes adjusted to the dark, I saw a boy about fifteen years old. He smiled at us weakly, raising his arm halfway in greeting, as if it took a substantial effort.

"Hi, man," he said.

"There she is," the girl said. She turned deliberately, as models do, giving us a show of her small rear. She pointed to a big, fat blonde woman sitting at the chrome kitchen table staring at the wall opposite. Her eyes had the torn, empty look of the person who is mad.

Oddly, she and the girl bore not even the remotest physical resemblance.

A tall, flabby man with a large pot belly entered the room.

The top of his face was strangely reddish, yet the mouth area was white, as if made up in the manner of a clown. He appeared to be blushing with half his face. He smiled questioningly.

Harry glanced at me, raising an eyebrow. A really weird crew here, right? Nobody in the family resembles anybody else. Nobody, I thought, belongs here. The man with the strange red face approached as if to examine me. I stepped back. He smiled as if I had answered some question he was asking me. He turned. He seemed detached now, indifferent to our presence.

"Well," Harry said, "let's get down to business." His eyes did a dying fall. "I mean, shall we just choose one or shall we take the identified patient?"

I ignored him and asked the girl if these were her parents. "I mean, your natural parents?" She nodded. Then, rather suddenly, she and the young man walked off quickly toward the rear of the house.

"Where . . . ?" Harry caught the inappropriateness of their action.

"Sir," I asked the man, "would you tell us how your wife has been acting?"

"Who?"

"Your wife. How has she been acting?" I heard the irritation in my voice. "You know, her behavior. We understand she chased a neighbor down the street with a board . . ."

"What?"

"He's hard of hearing," Harry said. "Among other things."

The man sat down suddenly, half in fear. It was all beginning to have that clammy, foggy-bottom feel. "Sir," I said, raising my voice, "can you tell us . . ."

"What?"

"Sir, can you tell us . . ."

"Jesus," Harry said, "I'll get the girl." He walked off. I heard some bustling and shuffling. The girl appeared with Harry behind her. She was buttoning her blouse casually.

Harry checked the ceiling again for help or clues. "Making out," he mumbled. The girl smiled.

“Damn it!” I said. “We have work to do. What’s going on in this nuthouse? Look, you called us, right? Your mother has been acting odd. So sit down, all right? We want to ask you some questions. And what’s wrong with your father?”

“She’s crazy.” She spoke disdainfully. “She chased a neighbor with a board. She would have killed her if she could have. She said that lady was screwing my dad.”

“I presume by ‘she’ you mean your mother. Was the neighbor, you know, screwing your dad?”

“Probably.” She smiled at her boyfriend. He grinned stupidly.

I approached the lady. “Ma’m, how are you doing? I’m Dr. Crain, from the Department of Mental Health . . .”

She mumbled some words in psychotic Spanish.

“Are you Spanish?” Harry asked the girl. She nodded. “Mexican,” she said.

“Were you adopted?” I asked.

“We are different from most people,” she said.

“Really?” Harry said.

Now the mother was hallucinating actively in the corner. She spoke in Spanish to the voices that were evidently answering her. The girl and her friend observed the woman clinically. The husband sat, smiling blandly. Harry walked to the telephone on the kitchen wall and called the ambulance. The girl sat on the arm of the chair where her deaf father was seated. He placed his full, flat hand on her leg, nonchalantly, well above the knee.

The woman spoke excitedly to her voices.

The thin, dark youth stood silently to the side when the ambulance arrived. The woman did not protest when we strapped her to the gurney.

“It’s a nice day!” the man shouted.

“I think I’ll skip lunch,” Harry said.

12

The supervisor at Human Resources had called the clinic for help. Harry became wildly aggressive at the thought of all those typists and file clerks. He threw his shoulders back, pulling in his gut. He was the attendant to emergencies.

He pushed open the large glass doors to the Office of Human Resources. He walked in boldly, leading the way. We saw three long rows of desks, perhaps seventy in all. Behind each one sat a woman, young and beautiful.

All eyes were upon us. We were the men in the white coats with the butterfly nets, there to scoop up some old man who had made vague threats to the women. And a flasher to boot.

"The County Psychiatric Emergency Team has arrived, girls. At your service. You name it."

Harry smiled broadly at the entire bunch. They returned his smile. A sea of bright teeth.

"This here is the doctor, ladies," he said, including me in the game.

The supervisor approached us. He was irritated, his manner fussy and effeminate. "Well!" he exclaimed. "It's about time!" He glanced disapprovingly at the women.

"Well, what?" Harry asked. "We got here as soon as we could, pancho. Where is our victim?"

"In there," he said petulantly. "That nasty man showed his *thing* to my girls." Inside the glass-partitioned office we could see the head and shoulders of two uniformed policemen and the head of an older man.

"You should have heard how he talked. It was *terrible.* He wanted money. He thought this was a bank." He smiled slightly. "He kept saying 'Money talks,' " he continued. "Then he put his wallet to his ear—empty, of course—to hear it talk. Crazy old flasher." He laughed a dirty laugh and scooted over to a desk. "Isn't that right, Martha?"

"Did you get a good look, baby?" Harry asked, winking.

The police officers were relieved to see us. The man was short with white hair, distinguished-looking. He sat quietly, withdrawn, talking to himself. By his side was an expensive briefcase. The policemen, both young, leaned against a wall. They were babysitters.

Suddenly the old man jumped up. "Hey," he said, "do you guys like to *fish?*"

I observed him to determine if he was out of contact. One policeman turned toward him, nodding his head. "Yeah, I like to fish."

"Swell. Me too." The old man leaned forward animatedly. He was eager to pursue the subject. "Listen, I know practically every fishing spot worth a shit from here to Vancouver." He wrapped his arms around himself. "Bet you don't believe me."

"Sure I do," the officer said. "I believe you."

"Listen, you guys ever fish at . . ." He named several places up near Barstow. We all listened attentively. The old man knew what he was talking about. They launched into a comparison of favorite fishing spots and fishing gear. It surprised me, the ease with which the officers made this shift. They had entered the world of the fisherman. There are islands of sanity, I thought, good-sized islands within the psychic ocean of the insane. Right now the three of them were in a world that excluded me completely.

The old man drew a map, sucking on his pencil tip thoughtfully. That was important, sketching fishing spots for those guys.

"Pop," one officer said, "you know, this is really nice of

you. Showing us where nobody goes. Most guys would never tell anybody. I heard about it but never thought I would find out where it was. This is nice of you, Pop."

"I know!" The old man giggled gleefully. "I been fishing thirty years now. Ever use *water dogs?*"

"Water dogs?" I asked. Some delusion I never heard of?

They all turned and appraised me disgustedly.

The old man leaned back. His face fell away into a terrible sadness. He was distraught. "Doesn't matter now," he said. "Nothing matters now."

"Why?" The young officer was concerned. He seemed disoriented. Then he began to switch in. I saw that he was an intuitive interviewer. "Tell me about it," he urged.

The old man paused. Then he sat up alertly. "Listen, would you guys believe that I was down in *Mexico* yesterday? I flew down there." We all seemed to have the same thought. The old man really believed that he *flew* down there yesterday without an airplane.

The supervisor had been standing in the doorway. He held a dollar bill up to his ear. "Old man," he said, "you are right, you know, about money talking. I can hear it. Old George Washington is talking to me . . ."

The old man was thoroughly confused. He puzzled hard over this intrusion into his world. We turned as a man, angry at the supervisor's blatant cruelty.

"That was kind of chickenshit, wasn't it?" the officer said. "You shouldn't make fun of a helpless old guy like that."

The supervisor walked out in a huff. We waited quietly, watching the old man. He mumbled something to himself. He looked at his empty wallet. Time passed. Minutes, years flew by. We could practically taste the dry dust of the roads he had walked on. We tread on rocky, narrow paths circling a favorite fishing spot. We turn toward Mexico. There he is, somewhere on a bleak, white cement street. A slick Mexican is telling him that if he is to clinch this big-time American-style deal he has to give him a lot of U.S. dollars, as it is money that talks. Maybe somewhere in Mexico that dead joke is sitting. The joke that was on him and confused the old man. For the life of him he cannot get the punchline.

He looked up at us. He caught my eyes. The man was not insane. He was too sane to ask us to save him. We heard the siren of the ambulance in the distance.

"Listen to that siren," Harry said. "No need for them to blow that siren like that. Just trying to impress somebody." He opened the briefcase. "God, I'm depressed today."

The siren wailed in the distance. It was getting closer. Did the old man realize that it was screaming his name?

13

Her husband had called the emergency service. He spoke in the deep, resonant voice of a professional actor or radio announcer. His wife was so depressed she could hardly pull herself around the house, he said.

I talked it over with Harry. It really didn't qualify, but we were doing more of this "reaching out," as they called it. An opportunity to do a little preventive work.

A tall, handsome man met us at the door. He flashed us a big, practiced smile. His teeth were polished and remarkably even. His face was tanned and his dyed gray hair was starting to grow out.

He squeezed my hand enthusiastically. "I'm very glad,

very glad, you gentlemen could make it here," he said, casually brushing his hair back. "I can't *tell* you how appreciative I am. Isn't it a nice day?"

Harry glanced around the area. He shrugged. The man looked familiar. Had we met before? I asked. He was immensely pleased at the question. He tipped his chin upward just a notch, turning it slightly to one side.

"I'm in films," the man said. "Mostly bits. I used to get a lot of work."

"Have I seen you in anything recently?"

"Well, you know . . ." He looked down, with phony modesty. "You might have caught me on a recent *Police Story.*"

The living area was dark. The shades were drawn. It smelled vaguely of overripe oranges and nose spray. I glanced at the kitchen area. Dishes were piled high in the sink. A carton of milk and a box of dry cereal stood on the breakfast bar. Magazines and newspapers were strewn around the room. A large, open box of candy and several bottles of pills were on the table next to the couch.

A thick line of used Kleenex directed my gaze to the woman lying on the sofa. She turned over, greeting us with a weak wave of her hand. She smiled wanly. She was a big, blowsy woman in her middle forties. Her blonde hair was carefully arranged.

"There she is," he said. "Look at her. Just look at her. She has simply quit on me. She has given up."

She turned away in disgust, showing her husband her good-sized rear.

He began his narration of their recent difficulties. Terrible trauma mounted upon awful dilemma until it reached a pile so massive and absurd that I had an impulse to laugh. He was being sued by some crazy, litigious young woman who claimed he had tried to rape her. He had been involved in a traffic accident, and his wife had suffered a recurrence of an old whiplash. Then his lawyer had missed the first court appearance at the hearing involving the young woman. The judge gave him a ten-day delay. The lawyer was late again. Arriving half an hour after the lady had been awarded a judgment that amounted to the couple's entire life savings.

"Tough, sure," he said. "But not tough enough—not enough—to get *me* down."

His wife moaned softly. She turned to face us. "See," she said, "what's the use? What's the use? We've lost everything. Everything." She glanced at her husband. "Other than that, things are going along just fine. Other than the fact that we don't have a goddamn dime to our name, and John here hasn't worked in months, and I got this neck trouble . . ."

"Look how she talks. See how she is? She's a pessimist." He appraised her with distaste. "That's no way to talk, honey. There's always hope, baby. God knows there's always hope." He smiled brightly. "If I didn't believe *that,* why, I would probably kill myself. But I'm an optimist. I always look on the bright side of things . . ." He turned to Harry and me. "What do you gentlemen think? Shouldn't we always look on the bright side? Honey! Honey! This is America, baby."

Harry sat down opposite. "You're absolutely right," he said. "This is America."

"Right!" the actor said. "Right on. If I didn't believe that, why, I would probably kill myself."

"Crap," his wife said. "Everything has turned out to be crap."

"Look, honey," he said. "There is always tomorrow. Always. You know as well as I do that the old sun is going to shine tomorrow morning. I mean, so what if we have a minor setback? It's only temporary. That's not enough to get us down, baby." He turned to us. "Tomorrow is another day."

"Crap. I feel terrible," she said. "I'm depressed."

"Frankly, honey," he said lightly, "your mood can be pretty rough to live with." He turned to us. "It isn't inspiring, you know. What do you fellows think?"

"Frankly," I said, "I think I might get a little bit depressed myself, with all that has happened." And with your attitude, I thought. It's depressing the crap out of me just listening to you.

"I could get work tomorrow," he said. "Tomorrow. I could get a play in Chicago tomorrow. Or Detroit. I could land a job there without a bit of difficulty. If I had the bread to get there. Repertory. That isn't too bad."

"I hear there are a lot of unemployed actors around," I said, trying to inject some reality into the situation. "The valley is filled with them."

"That's true. But they have the wrong attitude. They let a few minor setbacks work on them, heavylike . . ." He glanced at his wife's prominent rear. "You have to think positively."

"Oh, God," she yelled. "What a pile of crap. I swear . . ."

"See!" he yelled. "See how she is. Look at her. Lying down after a simple little setback! She's lying down on our lives."

"She's sitting up now," Harry said.

"You're trying to get me to join you in that dark, silly mood of yours. But I refuse!" he said. "I can get a part in Chicago tomorrow. If only I had the bread. Repertory. Then a part in films. Then we're back on our way again. On our way, baby." He smacked a fist hard into his other hand and began pacing the room. His eyes were wild, glazed over. "Who says I can't pick myself up? Who says?"

He looked pointedly at Harry, then at me, as if he might attack us physically if we disagreed. I kneeled at the base of the couch.

"See if you can get your husband to bring *you* into the clinic tomorrow or the next day," I said softly. "You know . . ." I glanced at him meaningfully. "Make sure he comes too."

"Thanks," she said. She smiled broadly. "I feel better. Thanks."

He showed us to the door. "Jesus!" he shouted, pounding his chest, breathing deeply. "Jesus, I feel good! I'm glad you came! I think I'll fly to Chicago tomorrow. Repertory. Nothing wrong with that."

"Don't forget the airplane," Harry mumbled.

14

The clinic is becoming more established. That might explain the increase in emergency walk-ins. Perhaps it is the gloomy days of winter that we are experiencing. No, there can be a coziness to these darker days. The air is soft and cool and it feels good to be inside, if you have the company of someone who cares.

Spring and summer can be more depressing. People feel their loneliness most when others appear so happy and relaxed. It is at these moments, they will tell you, when they are watching couples laughing together or young people with their lives all ahead of them, that they feel angry, suddenly filled with hate for all the happy people, and realize that their life is over or that they never even lived it.

Some people fear that they will kill themselves if they do not have some love at a particular moment. These bouts occur during the night, generally. During the day there is work to be done, and work can be a lifesaver.

But in those hours past midnight a person becomes aware that he is absolutely alone, sentenced to the prison of that bed and the prison of that moment. It is then, the person tells us later, that he considers ending it all. He lies there, almost afraid to breathe, as if any action on his part might stir his muscles into a sea of uncontrollable, random activity, devoid of conscious will; as if his feet might take it upon themselves to walk into the bathroom for those sleeping pills in the medicine cabinet.

"This woman sounded desperate," the intake worker said apologetically, handing me the telephone information form. "I told her someone would see her on emergency walk-in first thing in the morning. She looks fine today."

The woman entered my office, talking animatedly, as if we were old friends.

"There are a lot of things—a *lot* of things—people don't know about birds," she said. She set her small paper bag down on my desk. There were neat little cut-out holes on the sides of the bag.

"Can I look at him?" I asked.

"It's kind of hard to see him through the holes," she said. "Anyway, he's a her."

She smiled at me warmly. She was an attractive, blondish woman. In her late forties, I thought. Possibly fifty. She spoke with the high, oddly innocent voice of a little boy and looked as if she had somehow managed to bring her childhood intact into middle age. Her eyes twinkled in that vulnerable way of the person unprepared for the pace of the modern world, someone who would be at home in a forest somewhere.

"I'm a dingaling," she said, as if to help me in my diagnostic appraisal.

"A lot of people are a little bit dingie," I said. "What brought you into the clinic today?"

"I thought I ought to keep my appointment. It is only good manners, wouldn't you say? So many people today are, well, rather gross and crude. I'm not into that, myself. I do get desperate. I was desperate when I called. So I'm here. I probably would kill myself except that my plants and animals need me."

"How many animals do you have?"

"Fourteen cats. Four dogs." She brushed her hair back. An attractive woman, I thought. Why was she so alone? "And thirty-seven birds in cages."

"How about men friends? Do you have any men friends?"

The mention of men seemed to frighten her. She looked away. Softly she said, "They scare me spitless."

I waited a moment. "We're not all so scary," I said.

She smiled at me. "You don't scare me. I don't know why. Anyway, I'm too crazy for most men. Really. They find me very goofy. I am, of course."

"You don't impress me as being all that goofy," I said.

She fingered her paper bag. It was neatly folded at the top like a child's lunch bag. She held it up to her eyes, peeking inside through the little holes. "She's still alive," she said excitedly, turning to me. "Isn't that amazing?"

"Was she injured?"

"Yes, she was. I found her right out on the street. See," she said, "little birds, when they are injured, they think they are going to die. That's the way they think. That they are going to die. So what I do, see, is I keep them alive with surprises."

"Surprises?"

"Sure. Surprises. Like I wake her up with my eyedropper. I feed her sugar water, and I wake her up when she doesn't expect it. Birds have to be on the alert at all times, you see. It's because of cats and dogs. Cats especially. They are ready for them, see, but when they get hurt they lose interest, and they think they are going to die." She paused. "So I keep them alive with surprises."

"It's strange," she said.

I asked her what she meant.

"The way I feel. It's difficult to explain. I feel I am running at . . . at breakneck speed, as if sanity were in pursuit. Does that make any sense?"

"I understand that you are living by yourself."

"Yes." She folded her hands in her lap and looked at the paper bag. "She has to have the safety of a cage," she said. "It's terrible to see a beautiful bird caged like this." A tear rolled down her nose. "She wants to fly so *bad.*"

"I know she does," I said.

"She wouldn't last two minutes out there with all those cats."

"I don't know," I said. "Maybe she would, if she got stronger. Can I take a look at your little bird?"

She glanced up at me coyly. She thought it over, puzzling the way a little girl does when she pretends to be a serious, worried mother. She smiled seductively. "You might frighten her," she said softly.

"I thought you said that little birds liked surprises?"

She giggled. "Did I say that? Well, if I said that then I guess it's all right. Go ahead. You can take a quick look inside."

I picked up the small paper bag. The situation had become oddly exciting, suspenseful. Of course I anticipated that the bag would be empty. I held the bag up to the light, peering inside the holes. A little yellow bird bravely returned my stare, its little heart pumping hard against its breast.

"Not too long, please," the woman said. "Don't look too long. *Please.*" She grabbed the bag from me, holding it protectively to her breast.

Little birds need care, I said to myself. I wrote down an appointment for her on a slip of paper.

"Do you like kumquats?" she asked, smiling happily at the appointment slip.

15

Harry flatters me today. "You could make it in the state hospital, Doc," he says.

"Well, sure . . ." I don't follow him.

"As a psych tech," he says, grinning. He lights up a big cigar. He puts his feet on the desk. "That's saying something, Bill," he adds. "It takes a certain . . . maturity—that's it—a certain maturity to make it in the state hospital, yessir." He puffs his cigar. "I'll tell you the truth, I miss it. I don't have any place to take out my hostilities anymore. My grievous pain. I miss all that bony-white ass I used to kick, Bill."

"You didn't."

He smiles wisely. "I'll tell you the absolute truth." He pauses, looking down. "I actually did involve myself in a little tangle or two, Doc, now and again. I'll admit it. You know, some asshole calling us terrible names. It don't matter if he's crazy, Doc, talking bad like that. I mean *bad.* Whole paragraphs, and you *know* he knows better. He is asking to get his bony ass kicked, Doc."

Harry sighs. "Later I quit it, after a time or two. It made me sick in the stomach. You could say I mellowed early. I got my maturity early."

We discuss the strange phone calls we have been receiving lately. A number of clinicians received a call from this man. That was the mystery, how he knew the various members of the clinic staff. Who could the mystery phone caller be? Harry and I secretly thought that some member of the staff was putting everybody else on. Maybe the job was getting to him. Our prime suspect was a psychiatrist who had called the PET office earlier in the month, pretending he was a sexually confused young man. I had taken the call, and Harry got on the extension. We bit, giving the young man our best words of reassurance, so we got angry when we heard the giggles of the secretaries in the background. But this particular caller was not easy to place.

"Hello? Hello?" It was an eerie whisper.

"Yes."

"Is this the West Valley Clinic . . . ?"

"Yes."

"This is me. It's the Mad Murderer!"

"All right . . ."

"The Mad *Murderer.*"

"So?"

"Aren't you *upset,* talking to a murderer?"

"No. If you are a murderer as you say, then why are you calling up a mental health clinic? Tell me that."

"Because I'm mad, like I say. Don't you people cure madness and insanity?"

"Well, yes. I suppose you might say that."

"You don't believe me."

"No."

"Listen, tell me if this isn't the laugh of a mad murderer . . ." The laugh was so obvious, so blatantly put-on. We understood the young man only too well. He wanted so badly to be somebody or something. Better to be a mad murderer than nobody. And we did not know if he believed what he was saying. Or what if, God forbid, he was telling the truth? I did get an address out of him, but it later proved to be a phony. He began to call us regularly, making us anxious, giddy, and oddly exhilarated.

One of our psychiatrists, our clinic resident actor, discussed the pretend laugh of the Mad Murderer, whom I had dubbed M&M.

"I once worked in a hospital out in the Midwest with a nutty chief of services who laughed just like old M&M," he said. "The same hollow quality." He tried an imitation. "It's hard to catch the emptiness. It's not easy to take yourself out of your laughter."

"Listen," he said, "let me tell you about this weirdo psychiatrist who was chief of services."

He was the chairman of the evaluation committee at a state hospital. A real sadist who enjoyed "testing" the stability of the patients when they appeared before the committee for possible release. Maybe the patient had been working hard for months memorizing the story he was going to tell the committee. Maybe he couldn't remember things too well, with all the medication he was taking and with all those brain-scrambling shock treatments they were giving him. So he manages to walk into the committee room without breaking into tears or grabbing desperately for the old hideaways, like scooting off inside himself and pretending hard that this committee will disappear if he ignores it long enough.

Dr. Weirdo, the psychiatrist relates, smiles his sodomy-special smile, and he waits. Nobody on the committee says anything. They wait. The chief holds all the power. The patient attempts to understand what is happening. He wants his release. He examines the evaluation committee. All strangers. Even his ward psychiatrist looks unfamiliar. The gigantic oak table seems to stretch forever. It reminds him of a glassy airfield and he can see where it falls off into space, where all the weird monsters are waiting for him with their mouths wide open. He mumbles something polite and respectful. It shocks him to realize that what he has said was evidently unintelligible. Chairman turns to the rest of the board. What? What? What did he say? Did you gentlemen understand what he said?

Now he leans forward, smiling his evil smile, breathing his

rancid, hot breath into the patient's face. It is raining outside, he says to him. Did you say it was a nice day? Is that what he said? He agrees that it is raining outside. It is not a nice day after all.

The chairman smiles. He is relaxed. Hell, this one is a pushover. I see here in your records, he says, slowly thumbing through the folder, that you have this fear of airplanes crashing! Is that correct? Tell me quickly! Yessir, patient says. Yessir. Yessir what? Chairman asks. Yes, *sir,* I have this fear. I mean I *had* this fear.

Chairman leans forward. Do . . . you . . . still . . . have this fear . . . of airplanes crashing? No! No! patient screams. *Are you sure?* Yes! Yes! Well, is it yes or no? Patient says, You asked me. Chairman says, Do you want to be released or not? Yessir. Yessir what? Yes, *sir,* I want to be released.

The chairman slowly rises from behind the table. He speaks softly at first, then louder, louder. What if, Chairman says, you are walking along this open street and there is nobody in sight, and this gigantic *airplane comes swooshing down like this?* He jumps up, spreads his arms, and practically flies across the table. Patient cries aloud, Why doesn't he want me to leave here? Does he want me to suck him off?

Chairman says, Bastard can't make it on the outside. Take him away.

"Where is this chairman now?" I asked.

"He was asked to leave. The new wave and all. They got him out finally, though it cost several people their jobs doing so. Last I heard the patient was still there. For a time he tried mastering his fear by becoming an airplane and flying around the place. Then one day he just sat down and quit the whole business."

Grounded for good.

* *

"Doctors!" Harry said. "Same as you and me only more fucked up. One got cornered by a patient back in the old state hospital, and he screams for us psych techs to save his ass. Shit. We come on running down to bail that mother *out,* and we don't see him again for weeks afterward. Except in the coffee room bullshitting the nurses, or balling a young lovely in the laundry room. Someone accidentally opens the door, and there is his white ass pumping his expertise into her fine honeypot."

He leaned back in his chair. "But I suppose we shouldn't bad-mouth them." Then he sat up, leaning forward. "Why not! Sons of bitches get four times my pay, twice yours! For what? Filling out prescriptions is what. They don't even go out on PET anymore. And it's just as well. They ain't worth a shit on a call. They dally around and I could get my ass killed. Like the time this guy was threatening us, swinging a jackhammer high over his head. And the psychiatrist walks right up to him and *talks* to him. And the whole time the doctor's *talking,* this guy's swinging it faster and faster, winding it up for the grand slam. Know what I did?" He shoots his hand to his rear pocket, quick-draw like. "Reached back like I had a gun, see. Then I said, loud and mean, 'Put that thing down!' And it worked." He paused. "But what the hell was that psychiatrist thinking when he went up to him like that? That he was a doctor and therefore indestructible?

"The God complex," I said. "Thinks he's a savior."

"I don't know about a complex," Harry said. "All I know is that bozo can't find his own ass."

One of our consulting psychiatrists from San Remo sauntered in. Not one of our favorites. He turned to me and asked, "What's happening?"

Harry grinned at my predicament. "We were just discussing doctors. Tell him, Bill."

"We were just saying how old M&M could really use a doctor. He's been calling again," I said.

"Him again," said the psychiatrist, yawning. "Sometimes I wonder why I ever got into this line of work." He paused. "I know one thing: I like the *idea* of being a doctor. I watch all the medical shows on television. Yes, I really do love being a doctor. I masturbate every night just at the thought of it. Especially when I watch *Medical Center.* I even enjoy the series about the psychologist." He grinned at me. "Of course, I pretend he's an MD."

"Fuck you," I said.

Our storyteller was in a confessional mood. For a time as a resident, he said, he used an older psychiatrist's office in Westwood, moonlighting it with referrals from more established physicians. This meant seeing the people they didn't want to see themselves—deeply disturbed, rigid types, old hypochondriacs and hysterical housewives.

One buddy dumped this paranoid lady on him. There he was talking to her in this plush office, smoking his friend's expensive cigarettes, saying witty and profound things picked up from older physicians, when she noted, rudely, the pictures of his friend's wife and children.

"Yours?" she asked innocently. "Yes," he said, "my family." "Rather young, aren't you, to have teenage children?" "Yeah." "Funny, I had the impression you were still single." Too late to change the subject. "Actually I am married. I was married when I was fourteen." "You're *kidding!*"

She looked at him for a full minute, mockingly. Only a well-put-together paranoid could look the way she looked, he said. "Fourteen, huh? That's *young.* Really young. Do you know their names?" Right there, he said, was where he should have dropped it. But some mad impulse kept pushing him on. "Are you serious?" he said to her. "Of course I know my own kids' names." He pointed to the pictures. "That is Ezekiel . . . and Efrom . . . and Eve." Think an old paranoid lady will let go of your balls, he asked us, when she has them cupped right there in the palm of her hand? A paranoid lady? Never. Squeezed. And did she have to practically roll on the rug, laugh so coarsely, and for so long?

And would you believe it, after all that, the lady made another appointment? He paused, reflecting. "Saw her for a solid year. Needed an ongoing case, I suppose. Also needed the money. Finally I couldn't take it. Had to either terminate her or fuck her. I wasn't up to that."

"Have trouble terminating?" Harry asked innocently.

The psychiatrist grinned. "No. For one thing, I really didn't like her. At the end of the year I told her I simply couldn't see her any longer. She came anyway, pounding on my door. She screamed at me, calling me names. She yelled to all the other offices that I had balled her. Wasn't true. I cowered in that big chair," he confessed. "Cowered. Sat there and wondered what proctology would be like. Maybe brain surgery. Almost quit the field."

"What's proctology?" Harry asked.

"Assholes," the psychiatrist said. "You deal with assholes."

"I could be a proctologist," Harry said.

16

I am getting uneasy about our increasing involvement with the police. On our last call we had asked the police to help us out. Two cars pulled up simultaneously from different directions. Four officers hopped out. They immediately gathered together and began talking. The police are an in-group, a club. When I talk to them they look at me with that irritated, impatient expression on their faces.

If we greet them in a friendly way, saying, "Hi, fellows,

how's it going?" they look at us like we are from another planet. Who are you? Why are you so enthusiastic, so friendly, so *childish?* They remind me of the tough kids in junior high school.

Yet most officers are slight of build. These are not the ex-tough kids from junior high. Who are they? I think many are those nondescript kids, the ones nobody paid attention to. Everything is low profile. Don't talk too much, except to one another. Don't smile. Don't commit yourself. We reach a hand out in greeting. Nobody shakes it.

Policemen, by job and by temperament, place heavy emphasis on maintaining *control.* They seem to believe in the power of the will, judging from my encounters with them on emergency calls and in private therapy. They seem to equate mental disorder with weakness. Many of them become outraged at human weakness. They, like most normal people, project their own forbidden impulses onto others, living in the safety of the not-me. They act *out,* not in.

Sometimes they remind me of young boys about to act out a fantasy of war and devastation, like pouring gasoline on an ant hill. Only now that ant hill is this little house that we are walking toward, and there is this crazy guy inside . . .

The most awful things—like the Vietnam war—are viewed as child's play, events we only imagined, or events that don't count once ended. Life is viewed as a movie that can be run backward, or speeded up, or edited to suit. Maybe we are all losing our capacity to distinguish illusion from reality.

17

A volunteer from the valley hot line called to report a young woman who phoned last night while she was on duty.

"She seemed very agitated," the woman told me. "That's the dangerous time, you know."

"You sound like an expert. Are you in the business?"

"A professional? No. I tried to kill myself a couple of times." Her voice is calm, matter of fact. "I suppose you could say I'm knowledgeable in the area. Can you do something for her?"

I said I would accept responsibility for the young woman, not knowing what I meant by that exactly. I called the number she had given me. No answer. An hour later I called it again. Still no answer. It began to bug me. I saw images of a young woman lying dead on the floor or lurching about the apartment, trying to vomit into the toilet. Anxiously I paced the hallway. I kidded with the secretaries. Harry was out on a call with Al Johnson. I answered the telephone. Finally I had to move. I climbed into my old Kharman Ghia and headed for the address. None of this was according to the book. Technically we were not to make calls by ourselves. With those calls involving the opposite sex, a woman was supposed to accompany the team, though we frequently ignored this rule.

I inched my way down the busy street, watching the activity of the Valley upper middle class. Well-kept older women dressed in chic sport clothes meandered along. Self-important men drove past me, checking to see if anyone noticed their fancy Mercedes and Porsches.

My palms were moist. Why didn't the cars move faster? I began to worry about what I would find. Jesus, maybe I would be a suspect in a murder. I decided I had been seeing too many movies. I arrived, finally, in front of a large apartment complex. They were digging up the street in front. I had to drive around the block in one-way traffic. It seemed they were ganging up on me. I checked my watch. What difference did that make? She had had all night to kill herself. It was probably a false alarm anyway. I parked the Ghia in a no-parking area. Maybe I could explain my mission.

A tall, thin, pretty girl answered the door. Her face was pockmarked from a bad case of acne in adolescence. She appeared sleepy, indifferent to my presence. She was dressed in a long, dark blue housecoat.

"I'm Dr. Crain." I handed her my card.

She held it to her side, not reading it. Was she drugged?

"I'm from the Department of Mental Health. We received a call from a woman who works at the valley hot line."

"Yes," she said. She opened the door. "Do you want to come in?"

She beckoned me to sit. The room was tastefully furnished. Two chairs of Brazilian leather were placed opposite a long sofa covered in a light-colored suede. She sat deep into a chair and stared at me. I couldn't decide whether she was under the influence of drugs, in marginal reality contact, or simply a strange young woman.

Her hands moved about her face as if she were not sure the face was her own. Then she cradled her head, leaning forward, placing her elbows on her knees. Her eyes were an unreal blue, the color of faded denim. She had a square jaw. There were deep pockmarks on her lower cheeks near her mouth. She said her name was Betsy Ingram. She was twenty-two.

She spoke in a matter-of-fact voice, as if she were telling

me a recipe. "I simply want to kill myself," she said. "I'm not worth anything. It really doesn't matter." She could have been talking about an old bottle, a box of wet matches.

"I don't know if I will do it or not." She smiled at me. "It takes a certain courage, you know."

She had that hungry look of potential suicides. It is as if they cannot wait to make a meal of themselves.

I said the obvious. "Why do you want to kill yourself?"

She shrugged. "I don't know. I don't have any reason for living. If I could find a reason to live maybe I would want to." She seemed interested in the dialogue.

"Reasons," I said. "How can we talk about reasons? We live . . ."

"Are you an Indian?" she asked. "You look like an Indian."

"I'm half."

How disturbed was she? I couldn't decide. Her verbal associations were not unduly loose or disorganized, yet she did seem detached, withdrawn. And I didn't like that hungry, self-contained little smile on her face. I asked her to draw me a picture of a woman. I opened my briefcase and got out a tablet and pen. A man or a woman, I said. Either one.

"I'll draw a woman," she said. She drew a creature. It had a very large head and a scrawny body without breasts. It could have been a young boy or a girl. She had attacked the body with heavy, sharp lines like bent and broken knife blades penetrating the breast and genital area. The effect was shocking—there was so much self-hate, so much rejection of female sexuality. The face was sad. No, there was a note of desperation, even fear. The eyes did not see out. Rather, they seemed to be looking inside. A very clear and reliable diagnostic sign of extreme introversion, even schizoid withdrawal from the physical world around her.

She drew a boy. He seemed much healthier. His face was calmer, less tortured. His eyes seemed more interested in the external world.

"Your young man seems more interested and comfortable than your woman."

"I hate being a woman," she said, startling me with her intensity.

"I can tell from your picture," I said.

"You can tell that?" She picked it up. "Does anybody care? Does anybody care about anybody else? Is there any such thing as love?" she asked bitterly. "Doesn't everybody want something from somebody? If they say they like you they want something, isn't that true? Or even if they want to help you, it's their job. Isn't that right? Or it makes them feel good." She crossed her legs decisively. Answer that, she seemed to say. If you can.

She was asking the familiar questions asked by adolescents when they first weigh their idealistic values in the context of the real world.

"What do you do when somebody wants to check out?" she said.

I shrugged. "What can I do?" Those words—the flat, indifferent "check out"—made her life sound like something she could blow away like a piece of lint. I had been rejecting the idea of taking any action, but now it was all turning about. But what would hospitalization accomplish? These attitudes were relatively fixed for now. She would be released in a week or less. Well, if I heard that she killed herself later on, at least I would have done something. I considered hospitalizing her for my own sake, to get me off the hook.

"I don't want to upset you," she said. "It wouldn't be the world's biggest loss, you know." She fiddled with her fingers. "It's guys," she said. "It's definitely guys. If I could make it with men, I'd be all right. But all they want to do is . . . you know. That's all. I mean, that's not love."

"It can be." I decided I would not take any action. I would try to talk her into coming to the clinic.

"Do you want to know when I decided to kill myself? Last Saturday. I talked to this really cute guy who works in the gas station on Victory and Topanga, you know? I talked to him without shaking! That was Saturday. He was so gentle and nice. I wasn't scared at all. Then I went back. I didn't need any gas, but I went back there . . ."

She blinked her eyes. "Well, I drove up and I said 'Hi,' you know." Tears formed. "And he didn't . . . he didn't seem to know me. I mean, all that nice talk . . . he didn't mean it. It was just talk. It was just bullshit, you know that. And he looked at my knees, like he wanted . . . you know what he wanted." She began to shake. Her shoulders quivered. "He could see my hands shaking on the wheel. I held the wheel tight, you know. He could see how scared I was. And then I began to cry. It embarrassed him. He looked at me for a minute, and then . . . I think he went back to put his . . . to put the . . . nozzle into my . . . tank."

She breathed deeply. She smiled at me. It was a terrible smile. It spoke of resignation and hopelessness and a recognition of a crazy mastery of something that should never be mastered by anyone.

"So I just gunned my car and drove the hell out of there."

"What about . . . ?"

"His nozzle? It was still in the tank." She giggled. "It was weird, really weird. I saw it when I shot around the corner. That old hose was flapping away there like a snake gone nuts. Spitting gasoline all over the place. It was weird, really."

She looked at me pointedly. "I'm weird, aren't I? Tell me the truth."

I smiled. "A little. Nothing that a good relationship couldn't handle."

I wrote an appointment time on another business card. She looked at it for a full minute, as if deciding her fate once and for all. "All right," she said. "OK. What have I got to lose? Right?"

"Right," I said.

She eyed me distrustfully. I felt her anxious eyes probing my very being. I was being judged, appraised, and her life seemed to turn on the diagnosis she would make of me in the next few seconds.

"All right," she said, terribly tired now. "I'll keep this appointment. It can't hurt. I'll warn you, I've got some pretty deep hangups. About guys, mainly."

18

She sought to impress us with her toughness. She sighed dramatically, rising from her chair. "Getting old," she said. Her voice was low and harsh. She talked to an unseen listener to the side of us, but for our benefit. "These bones are creaky," she said. I caught Harry's eye. She had called us, but why were we here? She flicked the ash off her cigarette onto the rug. "Kills the moths," she said. She examined the cigarette. She reflected upon its length, its meaning in her life.

"Well, fellas," she said finally, "are you going to take her or aren't you?" She directed our glance toward the small kitchen area. We saw a slight, intense young woman looking at us with frightened eyes. Her daughter. She stood awkwardly by the built-in stove, shifting her feet as if she did not belong there but did not belong anywhere else either. Her chest heaved. She stood there a good fifteen feet away, though she appeared cornered. Her eyes darted from side to side. She wanted to run. I readied myself to grab her if she bolted.

I approached the girl. She turned quickly, putting a kettle on the stove, frantically busying herself.

"I won't hurt you," I said.

She looked at me inquiringly.

"Really. We are here to help you. We want to help you."

She opened her eyes wide, staring hard into mine as if she could not find me. She rubbed her eyes with her fists as if to press in reality. The kettle was steaming and hissing disapproval. She forgot the water.

"You need more water," I said softly.

She offered me a quick, tentative smile, her chest heaving. I looked at Harry. Do you think she's crazy enough to hospitalize? He shrugged. He didn't know.

Her mother leaned forward in her chair as I glanced her way. She was immensely amused. Patient in the face of overwhelming stupidity and incompetence, she sighed heavily. "Jesus, look at her," she exclaimed. "If that cookie has a full deck then I'm Queen Elizabeth."

"Come on," Harry said. "Be quiet."

She threatened to leap at him. She raised her hand half back. She wanted to slug him. Crown her, Harry, I shouted inside myself. Bust the old bitch right now.

She sensed danger and she sat back. "She does need help. Poor thing." She shrugged her shoulders self-importantly. "Christ, look at her. If that little honey ain't bananas then my name is Gary Cooper. *One* of us is out to lunch." She laughed long and hard at that one.

"Lady," I said, "your daughter hasn't done anything, you know. It's not against the law to stand in the kitchen scared to death and breathe hard. The law says you have to be a danger to yourself or to others . . ."

"Crap!" She stretched her legs out straight, taking a deep pull on the cigarette. "Crap, I say. You can see that little pussycat is zonked. You turkeys know what you have to do. I work for a very important man, you know."

"We know. High up in the state," I said irritably. Difficult to believe, but she spoke straight. He was the one who had called the clinic "requesting" that the team take a look at his secretary's daughter.

She blew smoke rings. "So you're going to grab her, or you're not going to grab her. Which is it, for Christ's sake?"

"We haven't made up our minds," Harry said. He gestured to me. We walked outside.

"I don't know. It's a tough one, Doc," Harry said. "Definitely borderline. We have to protect the girl's civil rights."

"Right. I only wish we didn't have that crummy politician in on the case. It complicates everything. I don't know what part he is playing in our decision."

"That old broad is a pain in the ass. I don't want to do her any favors," Harry said.

"That girl is out of it, though. She'll get worse if we don't move. I hate to just grab her. She's so scared."

"Scared of that mean old bitch, Doc. That lady is not in good shape herself. Why don't we just seventy-two that old white lady?"

"I hate to do it but I'm going to crowd that little girl. I hate to do it," I said.

"Right. Got to do it, Doc."

The woman looked up as we entered. "You guys better get moving. I got work to do." I wanted to shout at her that she was crazier than her daughter and I for one could see she had driven the poor girl out of her gourd with her phoniness and bulldozing.

She could not bear this any longer. "I'm going to get ready for work." She walked toward the bedroom, passing close to her daughter. The girl had been pacing restlessly. She turned away.

Suddenly I saw a handle and the flash of a knife. I froze inside. I gestured my alarm with my eyes. Harry didn't catch it. She stood two feet from me, her hands on the knife. I lunged forward. I readied myself for her thrust. She rushed right past me to attack her mother. I saw the mother's face. She was smiling even as her daughter raised her hand, ready to plunge the knife into her chest.

Harry leaped up, grabbing the girl's wrist. He wrenched the knife free. He held her firmly.

"She's not my mother!" the girl screamed. "She's not!"

"Of course not," I said.

I caught the look on the woman's face as I turned to call the ambulance. "Didn't I tell you?" she said, smiling. "Didn't I? If that baby isn't crazy, trying to stab her own mother, then my name is . . ."

" Joan Crawford," I mumbled.

19

"I mean it's hot!" Harry says. We are driving back from a call in the northern section of the valley. The sun beats hard through the glass into the front seat of the station wagon. He wipes his brow. "I play a lot, Doc," he says. "You got to. You got to play. If you don't, you might end up like that crazy old white lady we just saw."

We are measuring ourselves against the people we must deal with. How crazy are we? How *do* you keep your balance in these times? It is Harry's idea that you have to play, in much the same way a child plays, but you must know you are doing it. It is a matter of realizing you never really grew up. That is the key.

We also decide it is important to be able to put yourself in the other person's shoes, even somebody who is crazy as hell, in order to be sane, more or less. It is very important not to set yourself apart from your fellow man, or get too big for your britches. Harry says this is why the black man has the edge over the white man. He has fewer misconceptions regarding his worth. Serves you white people right, Harry adds. He shakes his head. The last call was a rough one.

I mention Carl Jung's description of a meeting with an American Indian chief in the Southwest years ago. The chief told Dr. Jung that it was obvious that the white man was mad. He did not *see.* The white man was always looking off somewhere, into the distance. You could see it in his face, that he was mad, the way he did not see. And he was mad because he did not accept the fact that the sun was a god. Anybody knew that.

Harry laughs. "Can't play, looking into the future like that," he says. "Can't be done."

*   *

We knew she was going to the hospital the moment we walked up the pathway to the house. Piled high on the front porch were torn photographs, broken frames, letters. She had emptied her life there, puked out all the mementos, the memories. She tore the sockets from the walls so the CIA couldn't hear their private conversations. They didn't need those walls any longer. Everything in the house was outside now. People could see in. No home now. No private places.

Once her sons had come running up this walk after school, happy to see her. She smiled. She hugged them and gave them graham crackers and milk. She worried with her husband about his failure to get his promotion. She was the strong one. Do this, do that. She wasn't much for feelings or sentiment. Now, standing outside on the street under a big fir tree, the husband told us how it was.

"I don't know what happened," he said helplessly. Was it him? Her? It all began well. Maybe she was a little dominant, but then he rather liked it that way—until it got out of hand. Why did she have to know everything, to control everything?

She began checking the locks on the doors at night. Then

double-checking. Restless, she wandered around, twisting the doorknobs. He buried his head in the covers. Is it really happening? Is my wife Margy going crazy? What could he do? People got better sometimes on their own. She refused a psychiatrist. Then she coarsened, got tough, more opinionated. She got angry for no reason. Flared up. Raised her fists over her head. She stared at him as if he were a stranger. Once she asked, "Who *are* you anyway? Do I know you?" Yes, he said, you know me. But he knew better. She was leaving the scene. He didn't know *her* anymore. She talked to herself all the time. At night she would turn to the side quickly, listening. What did she hear? When was the moment he decided to say to himself, My wife is insane?

The boys, all grown men now, looked at the floor, ashamed, then matter of fact. They cried for this woman, their mother. This mad creature scrambling around tearing out the wires from their outlets, her hands bleeding. This house looked familiar but it was nobody's home any longer.

The father stared at a flat spot on the wall. "I don't know what happened." He wrung his hands.

The ambulance drove up. We wrestled her inside. It drove away. "Well," the man said to nobody special. "Well . . ." He shrugged helplessly.

20

Harry and I were called to evaluate a young adolescent. Harry maneuvered the car up a winding road to the farthest reaches of the San Fernando Valley.

The summer sun had let up some in the past few days. There was a slight breeze and the air was clear.

"The man sounded cold, Doc," Harry said. "I didn't like him. He ordered me around. You know how they are."

I knew. We fancy ourselves as becoming expert telephone diagnosticians. You can tell a great deal about the person from his or her telephone attitude, from the first utterances. Some people treat us as if we are servants or lesser mortals. The so-called successful seem to be the worst.

We pulled up beside a gigantic brick home set into the hill overlooking the entire valley.

A fragile little man opened the door and silently beckoned us inside. He appraised us boldly as we walked past him into the vast living area.

The stone fireplace was ten feet wide at the base. It climbed high to the ceiling. The shiny oak and maple furniture was showroom new. A white baby grand piano dominated the far corner. A fifteen-foot sliding glass wall pulled our gaze outward to a long expanse of perfect green lawn. An oversized pool glistened in the sun.

"Wow! Some place you have here," Harry said. He was not impressed.

"Do you really like it?" The husband's voice squeaked behind us. He was a small man, almost dainty. He was groomed meticulously. His fingernails were manicured. He wore shiny red leather shoes with small string bows on the top. There was something oddly obvious about him.

"Sit here," he said, pointing to two rich-textured sofas grouped around the huge fireplace. "I'll get the boy."

We heard tinkly, tentative notes from a piano. It had the tinny, eerie quality of an instrument being played far off somewhere. The man returned without the boy. "My wife plays very well, don't you think?"

"Not bad at all," Harry said. His mouth was set in a grim line. "I had a couch like this once. Classy stuff." He lit up a cigar.

The man stared at him.

"Where is your son?" I asked.

"In his room. The boy refuses to talk to us. It's terrible, isn't it, the way young people are acting these days? That's why I called you. Imagine, not talking to his own parents. There is no doubt in my mind that this is a real generation gap we have going here. You would think the boy hated us the way he talks to us. To his own mother he shouts obscenities. He pretends he doesn't know who we are. He is putting on a big act. He wants to cause us more heartache."

I knocked on Herbert's door. A sign said "Keep out—this means you!" At the bottom was a crude signature, and in small, almost illegible printing was the sentence "Everyone in this room is dead or dying."

I knocked again. No answer. "Herbert?" No response. Surprisingly, the door was not locked. Harry and I entered. A teenager, maybe seventeen, was seated on the floor, facing us, smiling. His feet were tucked under, in a modified lotus position.

"Hello!" he said animatedly. "How are you?"

"Fine," I said. "Fine. How are you?"

"Come right in. This is my room. Yes, this is my room. I presume you have been introduced to those two people outside. One says he is my father. One says she is my mother."

"Yes, Herbert," Harry said, "we met them."

"The man is . . ." He looked at Harry. "Don't you think the one who says she's my mother is a beautiful woman?" His face fell suddenly, as if he remembered something overwhelmingly sad. He narrowed his eyes and looked from side to side. "Shhh," he whispered. He beckoned us to come closer. *"Those people aren't my real parents, you know. They are aliens! Illegal aliens. Wetbacks."* He laughed at this one. "Worms, see. They wormed their way into this house. They have taken over. You notice they don't talk like people." Hate flashed across his face. Then he smiled, rubbing the back of his neck.

Harry moved to call the ambulance.

"Please don't go! They are aliens who have invaded the earth! Are you on their side?"

"Herbert," I said, "we understand what you are saying. Your parents did call us. But we don't have anything to do with them. Not really."

"But if they called you and you came, you're one of them."

"Crap," Harry said forcefully. "We aren't one of them. We're here to help you. Shit, man, we're your friends."

"Really? Listen, I'll tell you I could use a friend in this place."

I surveyed the room. It was the typical room of the privileged valley teenager. Several large posters of rock groups were pasted on the walls. There was a small KLH stereo system. A speaker filled each corner. Herbert owned expensive earphones and a good two hundred records.

"Boy," he said, "I'll bet I must have walked a hundred miles. My feet are really sore." He reached down to rub his foot. "Do you believe we are real, us guys sitting here?"

"Sure, man, we are real," Harry said.

"You guys are neat. Do you know that? You guys are neat

guys! Would you be my friends? Listen . . ." He turned to the side, as if he had heard something. He smiled. "Did you ever think we might be dead, maybe this was all unreal, like somebody was directing us from outside, like we are puppets?" He rubbed the back of his neck.

"Why are you rubbing your neck, Herbert?"

"I'm being controlled, see. They planted a mechanism. I'm going to get it out, though. They know my thoughts."

"Sometimes everything seems crazy, or unreal," I said. "A lot of people feel like . . ."

"Hey!" Harry rushed toward Herbert. "Is that *blood* coming from the bottom of your foot? Jesus, Doc . . ."

"Yes," Herbert said, "that's blood."

Harry reached and grabbed a foot. I looked closer. I gagged. The bottom of Herbert's foot was bright red, oozing drops of blood. It was rubbed terribly raw, the color of fresh beef. And worn almost to the bone. We looked at one another.

"Did you do that . . . walking?" Harry asked, gulping.

Herbert examined one foot, then the other. He seemed indifferent, as if the feet were not his own and it was all of little consequence anyway.

Harry was near tears. "How could his parents allow this, Doc? Why haven't they called a doctor?"

Harry rushed into the living room, outraged. He returned with the father, half dragging him. "Look, bastard," he said, "I don't suppose you happened to see your kid's feet?" He pushed the man's face down toward the boy's feet.

"Oh, my," the man said. "Oh, my."

Herbert smiled blandly. He looked sick. The piano tinkled in the background. He yelled for the boy's mother to come in and take a look at her son's bloody feet.

"Will I see you guys again?" Herbert asked, as they closed the ambulance door.

"We'll be seeing you, Herbert," Harry said, rubbing him on the head.

"That woman says she is my mother. Isn't she beautiful?"

"Take care of yourself, Herbert."

He waved at us eagerly from the ambulance as it moved down the hill and away. Herbert's mother stood to the side. She cried, and she said, "There he goes. My little boy. There he goes."

* *

Harry was bothered by this case. With all his experience, he is still not the least bit desensitized to human suffering. He muttered to himself and cussed out loud as he piloted the big car back to the clinic.

"What is with these people, Doc? They *seem* like good people. Phony as hell, but they look like they try to do what's right. How can you go for days and not look at your own kid's bleeding feet? Jesus . . ."

He said that maybe he has had enough of this kind of work. Maybe he ought to go into a business deal that is cooking. It would be a relief to get out of the people business.

"I don't know," I said. "I think you would miss all of this nifty fun, being a mental health cop. Look how you get to let your mean side out, Harry."

He grinned. "Me, mean? Are you serious? I'm a sweetie pie. I kiss my sweet face every morning in the mirror when I shave. 'Good morning, sweets,' I say. Anyway, I'm an American. Americans have no meanness in their bony bodies. You know that."

We discussed this tendency we have of projecting our badness onto others in order to maintain the image of ourselves as good. I told him of a young woman I had seen this morning. You could tell that she viewed herself as a "nice person" by the way she sat down, smiling demurely, folding her hands into her lap.

"What was troubling her was this recurrent image she had in her waking state. She kept seeing this big black Cadillac rushing toward her, threatening to run right over her. Of course it scared the hell out of her."

"I like Cadillacs, Doc. The Cadillac is a substantial car. I wouldn't want a black one, though."

"It was like a real accident happening to her. She even pictured herself sprawled out on the pavement, all bloody and torn up. You could see how she was being visited by her dark side, the shadow of her personality."

"A Ferrari is a good car . . ."

"See, her 'badness' was overwhelming her. It was pouring right into her consciousness. It was awful. I didn't know what to do with her. I referred her to one of the psychiatrists."

"That shows you have good sense, Doc, right there. It's important to know how to make the right referrals. I learned that years back."

"We have to get in touch with our dark side, Harry, all of us. If we don't, it's going to come rushing in and overwhelm us. This image crap has got to go. It's killing us as a nation."

Harry yawned. "My friend, the one with the business deal, says we can make thirty grand the first year if we hustle . . ."

"Of course, it didn't help this woman that she had visited a palmist a month ago. The old lady said she was going to get into some horrible accident if she wasn't careful . . ." I stopped at the faraway look in Harry's eyes.

"Wouldn't you think," Harry said, "that his mother might have noticed little drops of blood on the carpet, or on the bathroom floor . . . ?" He dropped his head. The job was getting old Harry down.

21

I can see the people walking slowly outside, sweating under the summer valley sun. Harry is entertaining the secretaries in the humid cool of the file room.

"Isn't that how it happened, Doc?" he asks.

"What? I wasn't listening."

"How we grabbed that .22 pearl-handled baby right out of that crazy guy's hands?"

"Sure," I say, though it wasn't like that at all. So far none of the "gun cases" that we all fear has resulted in any real shootout. A PET member in a neighboring district got his finger broken, and several members have been bitten, even one or two on our staff. There have been a few torn shirts, one pair of broken glasses, and some arms with bruises where terror-stricken fingers dug around reaching at random for some security in this world. Our badges of courage. We love to show these signs that we are able to hang in there when it gets messy.

"Wasn't I terrific, Doc?" Harry struts around the room. The women smile at his antics. He is putting them on. He is putting himself on. "Tell them, Doc," he says. "Don't spare the gruesome details. Tell them the whole truth. How fan-tastic I was." He rubs his stomach. "A legend in my own time," he says. "A legend in my own time."

Later we drive to a call that involves an adolescent boy

who is threatening to kill his mother. We drive up and find five squad cars waiting for us.

We approach a sergeant. He is talking to a woman. The boy's mother, we assume. "Hello," I say. "We're from the PET team . . ."

They glance at us and continue talking. "The emergency team is supposed to be here by now," she says.

"*We're* the emergency team, from the clinic," I say, more emphatically.

"They should be here by now . . ."

I pull out my ID. Harry is grinning. "Look," I say, "we are the emergency team. Look, here is my identification."

"Oh," the sergeant says. He examines the plastic card. "Well, I figure . . ." He still has not assimilated our presence.

Harry gives instructions. He and I will lead, following the mother inside. Two policemen should follow us in. But when we walk into the darkened room *ten* officers traipse in behind us, completely ignoring the instructions. The youth is sitting in a big rocker. The police line the wall around him.

He looks around the room. His eyes are wide with anxiety. Then he smiles slightly.

"This is *unreal,*" he says. "Am I on television?"

I look around the room at all the navy blue uniforms. The officers are standing silently, waiting for me to act. They don't have any idea what to expect, nor do I.

"Couldn't some of you men step outside?" I ask.

Nobody moves. The young man views me as the leader. He looks up at me pleadingly. I shrug. "Is this happening?" he asks. "Is this really *happening?*"

I think, maybe we should go back to the office and start over. I can share the feeling of the young man who is blinking rapidly now, trying to let in more light, more meaning, as disturbed people will do.

"Yes," I say, "it is all happening. At least I think so." Joke. I turn to the ten policemen for their appreciation. Not a smile. Not even a grunt. Maybe there is only *one* policeman there, I think, but he has been mysteriously fragmented into these ten partial representatives of himself.

I begin the interview, feeling their heavy presence on me. It is not one of my better days. I want to impress them with my psychological cool, but my voice sounds thin and uncertain.

"I saw this program on television," the young man tells me. "It was a lot like this. A whole mess of cops and . . ."

I decide, after the brief interview, that the young man is disturbed but borderline. Harry agrees. "We can go home now," I say to the officers. They walk out slowly. The cop at the end shoots me a questioning glance. You *really* know what you're doing?

As Harry and I get ready to leave, the mother grabs us. She looks up at me with glazed, foggy eyes and says, "He's going to kill me, you know. I can feel it. If you let him go then my blood is on your hands."

"Well," I say feebly, as I close the car door, "that's . . . the way it goes . . ."

Harry laughs.

"Turn the channel and head home," I say.

"My blood is on your hands!" she screams as we drive away.

22

He knew the law and the terminology. He said his wife was a distinct danger to herself and to others. Would we come over and make an evaluation? She had purposely driven his official Cadillac off a steep embankment. She had ruined the car, he said, but only bumped her head. I thought he sounded disappointed. As they pulled her from the wreckage, she had screamed that next time she would do it right. He added, wryly, that maybe she was sore at him. Possibly, he said softly, he had been a little indiscreet at times, but why did she have to get so dramatic?

And how in the hell was he going to write off the car without the supervisors getting on his ass? Jesus, he said, how could she do this to him in these times, with all this accountability crap going on, when everybody and his brother thinks he is Ralph Nader?

His house was surprisingly modest considering he was high up in county service. The lot next door was vacant. You could tell a house had been there once, but the earthquake had leveled it completely.

We sauntered up to the official's front door and knocked assertively. A big, shapely bleach-blonde opened the door. You could tell she drank too much. Big red blotches showed through her heavy makeup. Her blouse was partially unbuttoned and her full breasts were tucked up under her chin. It gave her a breathless, squeezed-in look, as if everything were a constant surprise to her.

"Well," she growled threateningly, "what do you want?"

Her husband's head bobbed over her shoulder. He made foolish little pantomimes, trying to tell us to pretend that all this wasn't his idea, that we had somehow decided to drop in for a quick check on his wife's condition.

"Why don't you ask the gentlemen in, babe?" he said.

"What? Who? What's going on here, Bert?" She stood in the entryway unbudging. "Who *are* you?" she said. She narrowed her eyes into slits. We remained silent. "So what's going on, Bert?" she said again. She eyed Harry's briefcase suspiciously. She turned toward her husband with clenched fists. He ducked, feigning fear. I thought he looked like a drinker himself with his purplish-red face.

"Let them in, babe," he said. "These men are my friends. I asked them over. It's county business." He winked at us.

We grabbed seats at a table in the living room, off the kitchen. I handed her my card and mumbled something about being from Mental Health and wanting to ask her a few questions.

"Are you *kidding* me?" she screamed. "Are you . . . ? Jesus . . . do you mean . . . ? Get the fuck out of my house! Bert! Did you call these men here?"

"Dear," he said, "as a matter of fact, I did ask them here. It has to do with your attempt to take your own life, dear, you know, driving that county car over the cliff."

Her eyes darted from side to side. She began pacing. She was cooking up something. Harry and I exchanged glances. Would she get physical? What about weapons? She walked into the kitchen. I saw a sink full of long, shiny deadly weapons. She paused in front of them. Harry's eyes followed her every move. Then she sighed, changing her mind, and turned to face us. "Wow!" she said. "I can't believe what I am seeing here." She caught my eyes. She raised her eyebrows seductively.

She plopped down heavily on the couch next to her husband. She glanced at Harry. She held her gaze for a few seconds, then crossed her legs in an exaggerated, slow, casual manner, exposing most of a naked leg and thigh covered with varicose veins. She peered at me boldly.

"Haven't I seen you somewhere before?" she asked.

"No, I don't think so," I said, gulping. "I don't think I have . . . seen you before."

She grinned at my embarrassment. She switched legs with slow deliberation. Her husband shifted about nervously. "Dear," he said, "come on. Your dress . . ."

"Ever hang out at the Black Pussycat?" She turned to Harry.

"Never," he said.

"Come on, dear," the man said.

She looked right through him as if he did not exist. "Pricks," she mumbled, half to herself. "Walk in here for an evaluation. I'm going to give *you* an evaluation." She turned to her husband. "Big shot here," she said, "you probably think of him as a real big man, don't you? I mean a *real big man,* right? Know what I'm saying?" She grinned lewdly. "Not so," she said. "Not even close." She dissolved in tears. She began to narrate. Coldly, in a flat monotone, she spilled forth the most embarrassingly intimate and painful details of her life with this man. She droned on and on, her memory sharpening with each incision into their past.

She spoke of his sexual inadequacies, of hidden homosexual inclinations. Worse yet—much worse—she described intimate, happy, private moments, how and where they had first made love, what he had said to her in soft and precious phrases, what she had said to him.

Before our eyes she was killing them both by devouring the living essence of their past.

We listened, two voyeurs entranced by the obscenity of it, the methodical butchery we were witnessing. And it seemed necessary that we hear her out, as if it were our duty, having unwittingly participated in her violation.

Harry shuffled about. He had had all he could take.

"Lady," he said, "we got to go now. Right, Doc?"

Her husband looked at us inquiringly. "But she . . ."

"She's not a danger to herself or others, sir," I said. "Not right now."

"But what about . . . ?"

"We have to stick with our impressions at the time of the evaluation, and right now this lady is not in danger to herself or to others . . ."

"Couldn't you let them decide that at the hospital?" He was irritated. "After all, you're not psychiatrists . . ."

"Sir," I said, "that's the way it is."

"So if she kills herself . . ."

"I know. Her blood will be on our hands." This was getting old.

Later the husband called. He spoke softly, with obvious embarrassment, of their marriage, their early years together. They had been childhood sweethearts. Somehow everything had begun to fall apart. He had become an important man. There were other women. What is the answer? he asked. And what if she killed herself? I told him we were caught up in the way the law read. We couldn't hospitalize somebody for threatening suicide, could we? I added, cruelly, when I thought about it later, that she was pretty rational, wasn't she? I mean, her memory and all that?

He zapped me back as if it were automatic with him. "Incidentally," he said, just before he hung up, "she plans on suing you for illegal entry."

"Thanks," I said, "thanks a lot."

23

Obviously, observing the actions of people in their home settings is different from seeing them in the office. The office is the clinician's territory. People enter that territory with certain reservations regarding their conduct. In the safety of their homes, when company has gone, they drop all pretenses. To the clinician, practiced only in observing people in the office, seeing them at home can be startling. The real reasons for the person's troubles are only too clear.

Insanity observed on the home front is also more disturbing. Home-centered as we tend to be, we find the normality of a home gone askew particularly upsetting.

Harry and I visited an impressive home on the western edge of the valley. We were answering a call from an older woman. She let me know immediately that she was a very important woman with many influential friends in high places.

"How can we help you, lady?"

"It's my son. He's too big to take care of any longer. I told him he would have to leave, but he refuses to go. I think he has lost his mind."

How old was he? Forty-seven. Forty-seven? Yes, and it was time he left the house and got out on his own, didn't I agree? Cutting that umbilical cord could be tough, I said. She didn't see the humor, if there was any. Her voice tightened. All he did was lie on the couch in the front room and . . . well . . . it was dirty.

I banged the huge brass knocker on the thick, carved door. We waited. No response. We banged again. Finally a petite old lady, sixty-five or so, peeked out. She smiled widely.

"Please come in," she said, examining us closely.

I surveyed the large, intimidating living area. Two gigantic Grecian urns were placed on either side of the entryway. An actual Monet hung on the wall.

"Nice place you have here," I said.

"There he is!" she proclaimed impulsively. She pointed. Some forty feet away we saw a man sitting on a large red couch.

"Who is your friend?" she asked. I didn't understand.

"Your friend here. Who is he?"

"He's the *head* of the emergency team, lady."

"He's black." She turned to Harry. "You're black."

"Me?" Harry said. "Black? Why, Jesus Christ! You're right, lady." He checked his arms to see if it were true. "Doc, look! I *am* black."

"Actually," she said, "you have a good build. About six foot, broad shoulders. I like my men to have good builds." She surveyed Harry's body boldly.

"About the call . . ." I said.

She turned to the man on the sofa in the distance.

"There he is. Take him away. I can't handle him any longer. He's beyond me, gentlemen."

"Lady, we have to make an evaluation."

We approached the man on the sofa. He was muscular, tanned, early middle-aged, overweight. His face was puffy. His reddened eyes darted from side to side. They narrowed into slits, then widened to let in more light. Clearly he was in some inner turmoil.

"Mother," he said. "Who are these *men?*" His voice was high-pitched, effeminate.

"I told you. I called them. These men have come to determine . . ."

"But who are they? What do they want?" He was confused. He sat up straight.

"Johnny," she said, "we can't go on like this . . ." She was flustered. "Look." She turned to me. "You must take him away."

"Mother!" he screamed. "What are you saying?"

"I told you it would come to this, Johnny. I'm an old lady. You know that."

"You're *not* old! I don't understand." He began to cry. He threw his head into the pillow.

"I am old, Johnny. I'm tired. Mother can't be your girl forever. I have a right to some life of my own."

"Yes. Yes, you do. I know you do. I know it." He pounded his fists on the pillow. She began to rub his back. Her circular motions seemed sensual and seductive.

"Lady," I said, "what's going on?"

She continued her kneading motion. "He is my pride and joy. You are, Johnny. I mean it. But you are too much for me now. You must take him away. He isn't right in the head."

Her son sat upright suddenly. "Mother!" he screamed. "They're here again. They're here!"

I approached the couch. He recoiled in fear. He turned away, gathering himself in his arms. Harry caught my glance. He was hallucinating. Harry headed for the telephone.

"It's out of order," the lady said. "Nobody can call out."

"Lady, how can we make our call?" Harry asked.

"Go next door, of course."

He walked off angrily. She walked away. Suddenly I realized I was terribly alone. The man rolled over on the couch. He was caught in his blanket. He struggled to free himself, a big, red-skinned, thrashing infant. He rolled around, moaning loudly. The house was very quiet. The heavy luxury of the place weighed on the situation.

The man sat up. He was naked except for a pair of jockey shorts half hidden under a roll of fat. He was eying me now, breathing heavily. He raised an eyebrow. An overture. Where in the hell was Harry?

He leaped up. He stood, defiantly, not a foot from me. His unseeing eyes stared directly into mine. I could feel the musk of his sweat. Oddly, the old joke about Pierre and the moose call came to my mind. "Whatever you do, run like hell." Cool it, moose, I thought. Cool it. What to do? Should I just hit him on the nose and run? He stood there breathing hard, smiling a ridiculous flirtatious smile. I began to calm down. He hadn't attacked me yet. He rocked back and forth from one foot to the other, breathing heavily.

"Why don't you sit down?" I said, trying to be authoritative. My voice sounded thin. "Come on," I shouted, "sit down!"

He took a step toward me. Then, as if he had just been knocked silly, he grabbed the back of his head and lurched over, collapsing heavily on the couch. The phone rang. I could barely lift the receiver.

"Doc, Doc," Harry whispered. His voice was taut and strained.

"Harry? What?"

"Doc, now don't get excited. Humor the guy, Doc. The deal is, the bastard collects *guns.* He has a loaded Luger in there somewhere. A neighbor saw him with it last night."

"Swell," I said. "That's really swell."

"I'll be right over. I called the police."

I glanced at the front door. Then I had a strange sensation. I experienced myself running, flying, through that door. The intensity of the threat to my life transformed the entire situation.

The man rolled on the couch as if in pain. He moaned like a hurt animal. He grabbed his penis. More moaning. He rubbed his penis hard with the heel of his hand. I watched, fascinated. He had no erection. More rubbing. Sees himself in the feminine role, I thought. My analytical attitude calmed me. He grinned his goofy smile at me. His mouth was wet.

Harry walked in hurriedly. "Jesus, Doc, I didn't know. I

wouldn't have left you . . . What the hell is he *doing?*"

"He's masturbating."

Harry shook his head. We watched, captured by the gross sensuality. It was all so open, so public. There was a secret wonder to it. He increased his pace. His excitement mounted. We turned away. The orgasm was his business.

We stood there subdued, respectful of sex, of madness. The man puzzled at the semen on his thigh. Dutifully, like a good boy, he began to wipe himself.

Harry showed me the Luger. He had found it on the grass outside. It is a frightening weapon at first glance. But this one was made of plastic. It was a child's toy.

24

I took the phone. "Please," a soft voice said, "please come out, won't you? I'm afraid."

She said her husband was threatening to beat her up. He was losing control of himself.

"I'm not sure," I said, hesitating. "It's definitely a borderline situation. You can always call the cops."

"No," she said. "I think he's losing it, really."

"Won't he come into the clinic on his own?"

"No. He doesn't want to associate with all of those kooks, he said." He was an ex-police officer.

"Woody still thinks he is a cop," she said. "He says everything is going straight to hell, but he isn't going down without a fight." Woody had yelled at a youth to slow down as he sped down the street in front of his home. The kid gave him the finger, which enraged him. When he turned his car around, the older man placed himself in the center of the street, shaking his fist, challenging him to run him down.

We parked the car on the sloping grass of an unpaved street in the poorer section of the valley. Little Chicano and black children played in the middle of the street. The sign on the mailbox said "Dilworth Woodson." His house was a small, boxy white stucco set well back from the road.

"Old Woody has probably seen better times," Harry said. "Or he must have been a really honest cop." He knocked on the door.

A tall, broad-shouldered man in his middle forties opened the door wide. He was square-jawed, with close-cropped hair.

His voice was deep, authoritative, and frightening. "What can I do for you, gentlemen?" he boomed.

"Your wife called us," I said, deciding we had better play it altogether straight. "She's worried about you."

He looked us over. Surprisingly, he beckoned us inside. "I know she's worried about me," he said dejectedly. "I don't blame her. I'm worried about myself."

He shoved a big hand toward my gut. I stepped back slightly. He smiled a big, toothy, crooked grin. His mouth was filled with gold inlays. He smothered my hand in his, shaking it up and down. He repeated the same moves with Harry's hand, patting him hard on the bicep.

"I understand you fellows have a job to do. I was on the force for twenty-five years—vice for eighteen, narcotics for seven. I understand you fellows have a job to do."

His wife entered. She was a small, pretty woman in her early thirties. Her hair was prematurely gray. She seemed soft, rather fragile. She looked at Woodson with an expression that was fond and protective. The exceptional tidiness of their home drew sad attention to the sparse furnishings. There was a single chair and a cheap plastic-covered couch. An old Motorola television set played silently, the sound off, throwing a murky white light into the room. The living quarters of a depressed, impoverished man.

"Call me Woody," he said. "For Christ's sake, don't call me Dilworth." His laugh was loud and humorless. "Had to be a police officer with a name like that."

Old Woody appeared very weary suddenly. He sighed. He rubbed his hand across his forehead. "It's been rough lately," he said softly. "I think I'm in trouble." He pointed to his temple. "Mentally, you know."

"Why do you say that, Woody?" I asked.

"Fuck, I don't know. I can't be cop, judge, and jury, can I? I mean, I can't go around busting people, can I? I'm still playing cop." He winced.

"Well maybe, Woody, maybe you're upset about things, the way the world is . . ."

"Jesus," he said, beating his fist into his hand. "I would like to kick some *ass.* You know? Young bearded punks. They irritate the crap out of me."

He looked away, then jumped up suddenly. He paced the room, humming to himself, oblivious of the rest of us. I looked at Harry.

"You know what?" He stared at me in disbelief. "Do you know what?"

"No," I said, "what?"

He collapsed into tears. "I hit her, Doctor," he said. "Jesus, I never hit her before. It isn't like me. It's like . . . I'm watching myself do these terrible things."

"Sometimes," I said, "we have what we call complexes. It's like partial selves—parts of ourselves that we don't understand, haven't integrated." I attempted to explain with gestures.

Woody seemed bored, impatient. "I decided on my own to get some psychiatric help," he said. "But I just couldn't bring myself to do it." He thrust his massive chest forward.

"Pride," I said.

He nodded, staring me down aggressively as if he had to compensate for the mere mention of such a "weakness" as needing help for his problems. We won't hospitalize you today, Woody, I thought, catching Harry's warning glance. It would take an army to subdue this man.

Woody hummed loudly. He had zero musical talent. The tune was indistinguishable. It was a flat, forced cry of rage, I thought. His eyes were wild.

"I can't be cop, judge, and jury, can I?" he yelled. He had come close to a fight yesterday. He had accelerated his car and tried running another man off the road. All the man had done was honk at Woody impatiently.

"You should have seen his face." He flashed his crooked smile. In a way he seemed pleased with himself, with his fearless masculinity, and yet frightened half to death. The contrasting emotions could not mix into a single expression.

"Doctor, tell me, what is temper, anyway?" he asked.

I shrugged. I told him that temper was a complicated phenomenon . . .

He turned away impatiently. He wanted quick answers. "I got to whip this temper of mine," he said. "I could go to jail."

"Tell me a little about your background," I said.

He grinned. "It's interesting you should say that. Put it that way, I mean. That's part of my problem. You know, being a police officer for twenty-five years affects a man. It's a real ego trip. You're on stage all the time. You're right out there in the middle of things, and you're the star. It's tough to give all that up. I'm an egocentric son of a bitch.

His temper had screwed up his last marriage, he said. He feared it would wreck his present marriage. His trouble was he *had* to be right all the time. If his wife disagreed with him on some major issue, he was afraid he would drive her right out of his life. It had happened that way before. I said maybe he was reacting to rejection. What were the circumstances of his divorce?

He laughed loudly. "It was one year ago this month that my wife and three kids left me. I came home from work and the house was stripped bare." More loud laughter.

"What's funny?"

He stared at me. "Well, you know," he said uncertainly, looking down. "Look, I really want to whip this temper problem. Before I kill somebody." He cut the air in a karate-like motion with the heel of his big hand.

He had never had trouble like this on the force, he said. Went five years once without laying a hand on anybody. That wasn't easy. He knew of one officer who had his uniform torn every weekend.

"Policemen," he said, jutting his jaw out, "are an entirely different breed of people. You got to have the right temperament, though. I didn't. It was the tension. It wasn't that I was afraid. I had two operations. The doctor told me if I didn't quit it would kill me, so I quit. Went into business. Didn't get my retirement, either."

That was tough, I said. Didn't he even get part of it? No. He took all his money out and put it into the business. Then the business failed.

"That didn't bother me, though." He laughed his big, strained laugh.

"You're sure?"

He stared at me hard. His face squeezed itself into its fearless expression.

I told Woody to come into the clinic. There might be some medication that would calm him down. Maybe help him to look at the world a little differently. He seemed detached, sitting there, as if we had cut his tie to the world by getting him to talk about himself.

Harry and I waved at Woody, saying good-by. He sat on the couch, his big feet placed together, staring hard at us, his mouth pursed forward. He hummed loudly, waving his index finger like a baton, as if trying to recall an old song.

* *

"We couldn't hospitalize him," I said to Harry uncertainly, knowing he would agree.

"Nope. They would send old Woody right on out, Doc," he said. "He would beat us home."

Probably we would read about him in the newspapers. The pressures would mount. I could picture him trying to make a citizen's arrest on some muscular young guy. It would destroy him.

We decided that getting old in this society was a real drag. It was enough to make you dream up all kinds of compensating fantasies regarding power and aggression. If you were having trouble getting it up, you could always root for nuking your neighbors.

Harry surveyed the vast sprawl of the San Fernando Valley as we hit the top of a hill and headed down toward the clinic.

"It *is* a fucking movie out here, Doc," Harry said. "It is. Everyone in this whole fucking country is in a movie and we don't know it."

25

It was the brother of Alfonso Garcia, one of my regular patients.

"Alfonso!" he said breathlessly. "He's flipping for sure and he's dangerous. So what are you going to do about it?"

"Well," I said, stalling, "I don't know. He has a gun?"

"*Yes,* he has a gun. He shot it. What are you going to do?"

"What do you mean he shot it? Did the police come?"

"Alfonso," he explained carefully, "took his fuckin' rifle, aimed it at the ceiling, and shot it."

"No police?"

"Hell no! He was getting more impatient. The police don't always come, you know. They don't want to get shot."

Why did these Chicanos have to be so *definite* all the time? Any vacillation to them was like walking with a swish. "I didn't know he had a gun," I said.

I said I would make a home visit. I wanted to palm it off on the PET team that was on duty, but Alfonso was my patient so I couldn't get away with it.

Something must have been weighing heavily on poor Alfonso. Wasn't he taking his medication? At our last session he had become suspicious when I asked him if he was taking his Thorazine. His inner drama involved the great god Thor, who would zap him with a gigantic lightning bolt right up his rectum for all those terrible thoughts of . . . oh, God, he couldn't say it . . . of wanting to . . . you know . . . and wondering about how a *woman* feels when a man . . . and great god Thor comes out and zaps him. So don't ask him to take those pills with Thor written right on them. How stupid did I think he was?

So now he had a gun. It wasn't sufficient to do old Thor in, but it could spray his lieutenants.

Harry was off duty, so I collared Juan, a tall psychiatric social worker with a shaggy Pancho Villa mustache. "It's a gun case," I said. "Want to come along?"

"No," he said. "I don't care to be shot today."

"Well, *will* you come along? His brother hid all the bullets."

"Sure," he said, "why not? We only die once, *es verdad?*"

"What kind of character is this Alfonso guy?" Juan asked as we drove along.

"I guess we'd call him paranoid. Can't handle his underlying sexual impulses."

("I have a *girl* feeling, Doc. Do you know what I mean? I know how it is to feel like a woman!")

Alfonso lived in a crowded area in the northern part of the older valley. The houses were crammed together. A new chain-link fence lined the front yard. A sullen black dog roamed within, slinking about aimlessly like a caged weasel. The house was painted bright green, with yellow shutters.

We knocked on the door. Alfonso's brother met us and beckoned us inside. I brushed some stray Wheaties off a chair and sat down. Juan sat in another chair.

Alfonso walked in on cue. He was surprised to see me. "Doc?" he said. "Doc, what are you doing here?"

His father walked in. He was overweight and red-faced from years of heavy wine drinking. His eyes looked almost glassy. He was slightly cross-eyed. One glassy eye looked over my right shoulder. The other pointed vaguely in the direction of my forehead.

"The doctor just thought he'd come by and see you, Alfonso," he said, winking an eye at me.

"No," I said. "It's the way you have been acting, Alfonso. I heard you have been losing touch. You aren't taking your meds, right?"

"Doc," he said, "what are you doing *here?*"

His father was afraid. "The doctor just wanted to come over and visit. To see how you was."

I understood Alfonso better after this encounter. He was a victim of mixed messages. How could he possibly clarify the inside and the outside with a father who couldn't level with him at all?

I corrected him. "No, your family is worried about you, Alfonso. They called us. That's why we are here. How are you doing?"

He ignored me. He sat down at the table and fingered an open newspaper. "Look, Doc, I'm figuring out these words . . ." He caught my eye. He was frightened and very puzzled. "Look . . . see . . ." He had broken down the words in an ad, underlining some, finding different meanings, evidently, in new word separations and connections. Inside, hidden meanings were being uncovered. "Look," he said eagerly, "you think this says about the president. It doesn't say that." He giggled. Everyone sat quietly, entranced by his madness.

I remembered the gun. Juan had shifted in his chair. "Alfonso," I said, "you haven't been taking your medicine, have you?"

"I'm doing fine, Doc," he said. "Really. I'm doing great." His eyes narrowed and he smiled to himself secretly. He was scheming on the schemers. Suddenly he rose, startling us. He paced the room behind me.

"I got to get . . . an aspirin, man." I didn't like that "man" talk. I looked quickly at Juan. He nodded. Alfonso rushed into the kitchen. The gun? *Where was the gun?* Where was he going? He came back in quietly. He sat down.

"Who called you, Doc? My fucking father? My motherfucking brother?"

I waited for someone to speak up and be straight with him. His father stood quietly in the corner of the room shaking. He gave me a desperate wink with his crossed eye. Still trembling, he retreated to a corner of the room and waited expectantly. You are *asking* for your kid to hit you, I thought. Shape up!

"Fuck you, old man!" Alfonso shouted. "Fuck you!"

His father fell apart in front of us. He quivered. His head rolled around on his shoulders. Tears flowed from his glazed eyes.

"Alfonso," I shouted, fumbling for words, "are you angry at that old man there? What's going on?"

"Pop?" Alfonso shouted. "Pop? Hell no. That old man wouldn't hurt me." He ran to his father and embraced him. Tears flowed. His father tore himself away, dramatically. He cried along with his son. I didn't understand any of it. Alfonso's brother, forgotten amidst it all, also began to cry.

"Crap, Alfonso," he cried, "we all want you to get well." He rushed to join the embrace. The three then stood there hugging while we called the ambulance and got the papers in order.

26

She doesn't look him in the eye anymore. She doesn't squeeze his arm when he walks by. She rolls over in the night away from him. New positions now. He stares at the ceiling at night, listening to her whispers. Hurry up, old man. Hurry up and die.

"Maybe," I told his son, "he will have to be placed in a board-and-care home. Later on," I added.

I simply was not hospitalizing harmless old men today.

"Yes," the son said blandly. He turned to his father. They stared at each other. The old man was perplexed. "Who are you?" he asked, blinking his eyes as though he had a tic.

"If we place him in a home," I continued, "that will be the end of him. You know that."

"Well, he can't keep badgering my mother," the son said. "He's making her a nervous wreck. All that talk about sex and dope. That's ridiculous. Mother is not interested in things like that."

"But your father is not insane."

They had arrived, these good-sized men in their forties (the brother-in-law to help out), practically carrying the old man, who couldn't weigh more than a hundred pounds. He kept blinking his eyes, bewildered by this impromptu trip into town. They had told him he had to come down and tell these people about Mother and all the strange things she was doing.

The old man sat across from me now, low in the chair. He smiled politely. He did not understand why he should tell this stranger all about his personal life. He had probably decided long ago that he couldn't keep up with all these modern agencies. Here if you could believe it was an office where you came to tell some man about your private sex life, how your wife had become a crazy sex fiend and was having intercourse with Mexicans and niggers. But then maybe it made some sense, come to think of it. Maybe they could get her to stop. He smiled wanly. Where did you begin in such matters?

The son and son-in-law sat quietly, waiting for the old man's psychosis to show itself. Nothing happened. We sat waiting.

It took a single question to determine that he was not insane. Arteriosclerotic, yes. I shouted my questions. Hard of hearing, yes.

"Why are you here this morning?"

He pointed to the son and son-in-law. He was amused. All this modern-day fuss. The world had gone mad.

"What has been going on at home?" I yelled.

"What?"

"Your wife!"

"Yes?"

"You say she hasn't been acting right?"

We waited for my questions to sink in. Then he began telling me his story, slipping off the track as he went. His old circuits were shorted out in spots. He went along and then completely forgot what he was talking about. He dug around inside his head for a while, then brightened up. He had found a marker. Mainly it had to do with neglect, he said. Doesn't kiss him good night. Just lies in bed. She won't . . . you know . . . let him, well . . . Obviously something was up. It was the blacks and the Mexicans. And sex and dope.

Couldn't even pronounce "intercourse." He called it "intracourse." He laughed delightedly at what emerged from his mind. Imagine telling a stranger in front of your family about your sex life! In a way it was liberating. He enjoyed it once he got going.

"How do you know she is sleeping around?" I shouted.

"What?"

"How do you know . . . !"

"Eh?"

"Your wife . . ."

"Yes, my wife."

"Never mind."

I told his son that he was lucky to have such a fortunate example as this horny old father of his. He smiled indulgently. He considered me crude. Sissy, I muttered to myself. The old man talked on. He raised his sad eyes to mine. Eyes that told me his wife didn't want him anymore. As they walked out the door, the old man grinned at me over his shoulder.

"It's the times we live in," he said. "Mexicans and niggers. Everybody is sex crazy."

27

Summer has ended. The days are getting shorter. The trees are losing their leaves. The air seems softer, colder. We drive now with the windows up on the station wagon.

I watch Harry as he smokes his thin cigar with the attached plastic mouthpiece. What is he thinking now? One never knows for sure.

"You are an Indian, Harry," I told him last week. "You eat when you're hungry and you sleep when you're sleepy."

"I do exactly that, Doc," he said. "Exactly that." He grinned. He realizes his advantage over some of the hard-driving professionals. I am positive he sleeps in the PET office when things are slow, but you would never know it the way he wakes up immediately when someone enters. "Come on in," he says, busily writing on his scratch pad. "Come on in."

I believe Harry has found his way. I have run across a few others who have found their way. Musicians. An artist or two. Mostly older black people. They seem to walk differently from the rest of us. They *glide.* They are at peace with themselves. They have given in. Not up: in. Is this what is meant by having soul?

"I hear we are getting an additional psych tech position," Harry says. "This PET stuff is becoming big time, Doc. I hear they got PET in Orange County now. One PET man. He goes out *alone.* Can you believe it? He grabs some help when he can get it." He looks off into the distance. I can tell now he is leaving for sure.

*   *

Harry was intensely taken by this young woman who walked into the clinic stating that she was lost, man, really lost. He beckoned me in to help with the evaluation.

She was tall, with golden hair and a goofy getup. Inside the band of her floppy hat were .22 caliber shells converted into miniature vases that held little desert flowers in pastels of blue, brown, and pink. A single Indian feather was stuck in the brim. She wore patched old Levis and one-way dark glasses with big shiny stars for eyeballs. A space-age Orphan Annie. She saw us but we couldn't see her. No windows to the soul, but there was a lot left to see. The girl was truly attractive and shapely, but we wanted to see those eyes. You don't miss eyes very much until you can't see them. She was inviting us to examine her body while she watched us. She smiled that small smile of awareness that we were admiring her openly. It was a very erotic moment, being invited to do the forbidden. Harry grinned his approval.

"Hey, baby," he said, "where did you get that nifty hat? That hat is something else."

"Made it, honey," she said.

Harry slapped his leg. She smiled. Then she yawned without covering her mouth. She appeared tired.

"Have you eaten?" I asked. She looked hungry and she seemed fuzzy-headed.

"I don't know whether I have or whether I have not eaten," she said, removing the floppy brown hat. "Been on the road, man," she said. "Fucking truckers." She twirled her string of Indian beads, putting them in her mouth. She looked up seductively. Unpredictably, almost shouting, she said, "I'm a mark, man. A fucking mark!"

Harry and I were both caught off guard. "A fucking mark, man! I have hitchhiked all over this really *screwed* country and all I have been doing, man, is fighting off those fucking truckers, man. I mean it has been a full-time occupation, man.

"Listen, man, I'm not with it anymore. I seriously consider the possibility, man, that I am losing my *hold,* man, my hold. I'm tired, man. Tired. You could say this little chiquita has been on the road, and she is tired and dusty." She leaned back, resting her head on the top of the small plastic couch. She fumbled for a cigarette. Her hand shook as she lit up.

"Why don't you take off them glasses," Harry said, "so we can see you better?"

"Well," she said, "I just don't feel comfortable, man. I don't exactly dig it, you know, looking at this fuckin' *world,* man."

"Listen," I said, "tell us what brought you in to the emergency service."

"Got to have psy-chiatric help, man. Psy-chiatric help. I'm a basket case. Can't make it in this world. I admit defeat, man. Defeat."

She turned her head toward me, fixing the two large silver stars upon me, like some gigantic insect. Her mouth was set in a firm line. "Man, I'm tired, you know. I've been balling truckers from here to St. Louis. Tired says it, man."

"Easy does it, baby," Harry said, sensing genuine despair.

"Well, shit! I'm a mark, man. Wasn't I going to be a model? Then wasn't I going to be a starlet? So of course I became a *hooker,* man. I've done my share of jobs and I'm tired, and that is the truth."

"How old are you?" I asked.

"I'm nineteen, man. Nineteen. Been across the USA three times. What I have seen you wouldn't believe. Name it and I have done it. What I haven't seen hasn't been invented, man. Would you believe I was molested when I was five years old?"

We nodded.

"Five years old, man. That's pretty fucking young."

We nodded.

"By my own father, man. Now that is not right. And then I was molested again at nine. Would you say that was the right way to raise a child?"

"No."

"Do you want to hear how it was? I mean, really . . ."

"Well, we are on emergency . . ." I said.

"I'll tell you. To begin with, my mother is a bitch. A drunk and a whore. I remember coming home at night sometimes and seeing her balling some guy on the couch. And my dad used to drink a lot. It wrecked his liver. He has had ten operations, man. They can't operate anymore, man. Too much scar tissue. So you could say he has had it. I love him, of course. After all, he is my father. My mother is a lush. I hate her. Can you respect a whore, man? One of my sisters is working right now in Vegas, in a stable. Do you know what a stable is, man? That's awful. Wouldn't you say that is awful?"

We sat back. We were resigned to a lengthy narration. She droned on. From time to time she asked us if something was right or not. We had to answer the telephone as she talked on.

Emergencies. Mothers with sons who were going insane. Wives and husbands in serious conflict. A police sergeant called. On and on she talked. Fathers, stepdaughters, cousins who were really mothers of uncles, and stepfathers who were her sisters' brothers. Everybody was balling everybody regardless of age or placement in the family order. Intermixed were statements by aunts and half-cousins regarding the immorality of child molestation, or of fags and lesbians. Finally she arrived at early adolescence.

"I was fourteen, man, when I split. Ran away with this big black dude. Big as *you,* man. Hung like a champ. My parents wouldn't talk to me for two years. Don't see how my father had room to talk. Like I used to play games with him when he was drunk, man. Some games, man. Later on I told him that wasn't right, you know. He said I was nothing but a two-bit whore. That is chauvinism, man."

She described in pornographic detail her road experiences. She recalled every pass, every gesture. A gang of Mexican-American youths raped her. One of them broke her finger deliberately. She held it up proudly. She stroked her hips. I stifled a yawn. Harry's eyes were glassy.

"Look," I tried again. "Why are you here?"

"My social worker sent me over, man. She said I needed psychiatric help."

"Got to keep that social worker happy," Harry said.

"Right, man," she said. "Do you guys think I am crazy?" She looked at me with anticipation.

"A little," I said. "A little, maybe. But then, who isn't?"

"That's *right,* man. Who isn't? This is a high-flying ass, though, right?" She patted her ass lovingly.

"Right."

She giggled delightedly. "Do you really think I'm crazy?"

"Sure I do. Only a little bit, like everybody else. Just a touch." I twirled my finger at my temple. I made an inch of space with my finger and thumb. "This much."

She giggled.

"Look," she said, "do you guys want me to take off my glasses? I'll do anything I can for you. Anything. I'll be happy to accommodate you guys. You know what I mean?"

"No," Harry said gently. "We have these emergencies . . ."

"God, I could sit here all day with you guys. All day. I got more stories, man. You know, I like you guys. I mean it." Her eyes were moist. "I mean—how can I say it—you guys are a couple of swell dudes. Do you really think I'm touched in the head?"

"Yes. Yes, I do. But not too much. Just a little bit. And I should know. I'm the expert."

"That's right, man." She grabbed her sides. "Like, it's official, man. Listen, I have more stories. One time, see, I was in a gang bang, man. Boy, I thought they were going to kill my *ass,* man."

I ushered her out, gently. I told her we would like to hear more of her swell stories but the emergency service had to go on, you know?

"Hey, man, I get it. Like the postal department, right?"

She waved at us, sweeping her hand across the space between us like a little kid wiping the blackboard.

"Take care," Harry said.

* *

The days have been colder. Southern California does have its seasonal changes, but it is all subtle, undramatic. It is variable. One day the sun comes out bright and clear and the next day it is foggy and damp, threatening a rain that changes its mind, turning again into bright sunshine. Labor Day has passed and staff vacations are ended. New faces appear on the PET team. We are to involve ourselves in more prevention. I note new trends appearing in the fields of mental health and corrections. Psychiatry is under fire. There is talk of a "patients' bill of rights." Rioting in the prisons. Imagine, felons viewing themselves *solely* as political prisoners? Will the present conceptions and laws regarding enforced hospitalization hold up? We can verify the need for more treatment. Surely this has not been well thought out.

28

They were two round little people in their late fifties. No more than five-foot two by my estimate. He wore a checkered sport coat and a wild flowery tie.

"Are you a salesman?" I asked.

"That's amazing," he said. "Amazing. How did you guess?"

"Intuition," I said.

He told the intake worker it was a definite emergency. His wife was acting weird. He thought possibly she was possessed by the devil. He had read all about it.

"I'm Jewish," he said, "but it could happen even if you're Jewish. She really gets crazy." He pointed to his little wife. She sat on the couch, her feet barely touching the floor, idly staring at the walls of my office. She looked like a little girl who had been sent to the school principal.

"How are you feeling?" I asked. She smiled at me. Was she out of contact?

"So what do you think about what your husband is saying?"

She shrugged.

I turned to the husband. "Doesn't she talk much?"

"She talks," he said. "Believe me, she talks. What's your opinion regarding the probabilities of human possession? Is it possible?"

"I've heard of cases," I said.

"It could happen," he said. He looked at his wife. "Will she have to go to the loony bin?"

"We don't call it the loony bin," I said. "Do you know what day it is?" I asked her.

She shrugged.

"Where do you live?"

She said nothing.

"What month is it?"

Again, nothing. You couldn't hospitalize somebody for refusing to talk.

"I can't help you or your wife if I can't interview her," I said.

"Look," he said, "here is how she gets." He dropped down on the floor. He began rolling around, as if having an epileptic seizure. He pounded his fists on the rug over and over, breathing hard. Lying on his back, he stomped his feet up and down. He was making me uneasy. Was he the one to consider for psychiatric help? Medication, possibly?

He sat next to his wife, pleased with himself. Two round little people, sitting there, with feet barely touching the rug. After thirty years they were twins, practically. Maybe, I thought, he was once six feet tall, and he shrank to accommodate the relationship.

"I know how I am. I get myself all worked up," the woman said, startling me. "Something just comes over me. I can't help it." Her face began to redden. Her eyes narrowed. A slight, evil grin appeared. "I think," she said, "maybe I get possessed." She seemed to transform before our eyes. Malevolence grabbed her in its clutches.

"It's possible," her husband said.

What was happening? I stared at these two little people. They were grinning at me now. Two mouths smiled a single mischievous smile. I blinked. If this was a put-on, it was the best one yet.

"I don't know about all of this possession business," I said. I looked her in the eye. Her eyes were clear. She seemed alert. "You don't look crazy," I said. I examined her features. She appeared embarrassed more than out of contact. Ashamed. No, she was angry; that was it. I jumped in.

"You know what I think?"

"No," she said mischievously, "what?"

"I think you are angry. Very, very angry. That's what is possessing you. Anger. Sometimes it feels like that, when we're not used to it. It feels, well, kind of *demonic.*"

She grinned.

"You are a bad little girl, aren't you?" I said.

"I can't help myself," she said soberly. She was being adult now. "I think I am going crazy. You should see how weird I have been acting lately."

"Acting?" I asked. "Are you acting?"

She glanced at me meaningfully. "I've been acting crazy," she said instructively. "Sick."

"Acting bad," I said. "You've been acting like a bad little child."

"No, I'm crazy. I'm sick, really."

"She is really crazy, Doctor," her husband said. He twirled his finger at the temple.

"Have you any idea why your wife is so angry?"

He mulled that over. "Hmmm. I never thought of her as angry. That's interesting." He rubbed his chin. "She is sexier lately," he said excitedly. "I know that. Angry? Well, yeah, she is angry. She doesn't like me at home all the time. She says it is driving her crazy the way I hang around the house all day long."

"But what do you think has made her more angry than usual?"

"Nothing. Nothing I can think of. She has always been a worrier. The inflation. The prices. The energy. It's terrible how she worries."

"Of course I worry!" she shouted. She startled us again. She clenched her fists. She was furious. "Of course! Of course!"

She sat back, puzzled, disoriented. Unstable, I thought. No doubt about that. But not hospitalizable. What would that accomplish? I hoped she wouldn't get more dramatic. I began planning my strategy. Should I see them together for short-term counseling? They were a couple for sure. A set. One could not conceive of them as individuals.

"Are you retired?" I asked him.

He nodded. "We got less money coming in. I decided after my brother died of a heart attack that I was going to retire early. Why kill myself? Why check out before your time? So I retired last year. But with the inflation, it's all got her worried. She can't sleep. She says she hasn't slept in a month. She says it's a big conspiracy."

"She hasn't slept in a *month?*"

She shrugged.

"Really? You know you can get pretty toxic not sleeping," I said. "You can get pretty goofy just from fatigue."

"She's goofy all right."

"Don't you think she is also angry, having to worry about the reduced income and all? Maybe she is sore because you are calmer and are happy and she has to carry all the worries."

"So *that's* it," he said. "She is mad at me for getting to take it easy. But why should I go to an early death? It doesn't make sense."

"Your wife does all the worrying," I said.

He reflected. "Yes, I suppose she does. She always has. She enjoys worrying."

She glared at him, her fists clenched. He was pushing the wrong button again.

"Why should I suffer because she suffers and worries? Does she want me to suffer? Do you?"

"Damn right I do!" she screamed. "*Damn right!* Who wants to suffer all by themselves? Why should *you* get to take it easy and I got to suffer all by myself?" She began to cry.

"I don't think your wife is crazy," I said.

She was calmer now. She turned to her husband. Her slight grin said that when she got him home there would be hell to pay.

"Let's go," she said. "Let's go home. The man says I'm not crazy, so I'm not. It's official."

29

The valley area we cover is so vast that a call can be thirty minutes away, even going sixty-five miles an hour. Of course sixty-five or even fifty-five is a blistering pace for Harry, who drives like an old man with a year to live.

A big event in his day, I tell him, is when he negotiates the big county wagon around a stalled truck on an empty street. Harry cannot easily talk and drive at the same time. With half of a story to go and approaching home base he will slow the car to a crawl. He synchronizes his speed with the time he will need to finish his story. Once he stopped dead in traffic in order to apply the final touches. Another time he got so wound up in what he was saying that he completely forgot an emergency call.

It is a dreary fall day. The weather has been weird lately.

First it rains for a week and floods the streets, then the sun comes out and it is hot, and then it is misty and overcast for days.

"What do you think about all this people scooping?" Harry asks.

I tell him I am still making up my mind. That is partly why I am writing about it. You get to know what you think when you write about it.

"I am going to give it up, Doc," Harry says.

Our eyes meet. What can you say?

"Phasing it out, Doc," he says. "Phasing it out. This call here makes me think this is where I came in, anyway."

* *

We were off again to visit the M.P.'s scrawny mother. This time we were chasing her into a parking lot with skip loaders and lawn mowers running interference. And even as she cowered behind a tool shed, I was checking out the equipment there in case I needed to rent something someday.

What was I doing here, gasping for air, chasing this woman down a gravel alley behind a bunch of red and white trucks?

I saw her peeking out from behind the shed. Harry was circling the lot, sneaking up on her. Who was crazy here? What in God's name was I *doing* here?

Why did the son have to find her again? Why couldn't he just leave his mother to heaven, or oblivion? I mean, I was getting too old to chase around the valley like this. "My mother is starving to death," he had said. "Please come!"

There she goes! Obviously has some energy left in her. Here comes her plodding middle-aged son. Face wet with tears, heading her off at the pass.

Well, we had her again. She was standing not three feet away. Breathing so hard I feared she might have a heart attack. Frightened little bird, slacks all wet, scrawny chest heaving away. Please don't be so frightened, lady! Harry, let's forget the whole thing. Let's take her home and feed her. Feed her on a high-protein diet. Tiger's milk. She'll be out in another two weeks, anyway. Let's let her go.

Harry lifted her up from the waist. Threw her easily over his shoulder. She screamed that scream again! "May God rebuke you!" I thought I saw dark rain clouds begin to part and a giant hand reach out to squash me. And her eyes . . . those eyes, as they drove off in the devil's chariot. I still see those eyes.

30

Some people we see do not appear to have any core, any real substance to their being. They seem to exist as semantic constructions.

An attractive brunette walked in. In a flat, unemotional voice she spoke of herself as if she did not exist in a physical sense. She talked all *about* herself, surrounding her emptiness with so many cluttered words. I suppose this means I am this kind of person, she said. Or that means I am that kind of person. She was this; she was that. Defined by the words of others as she imagined them evaluating her. Where was her center, her being?

Then a strange little man walked in. Surely he had no center. His name was Demarco. He entered my office half shouting his words, as if he lived within his angry sentences. He seemed to be intent upon convincing himself that he was a fierce individual, unafraid of these doctors here.

Mr. Demarco had no idea who or what he was. He seemed to believe that others might let him know after he put on his act.

What will happen to the inner self if we insist upon "being for others" and not for ourselves? Isn't it likely we will then lose our centering capacity by default? Without knowing who we are, we are free to consider alternative selves. If we can be any number of who's, why not be one that is exciting, or even dangerous, like Mr. Demarco here? Surely then we will get some response from others.

"If something isn't done right away about my brother, then I'm the one who is going to kill somebody!" he yelled. "I mean it." He paced the floor. He pierced me with his eyes. "I'm going to get guns, see, or bombs, or something. Tanks. I mean it. My poor brother." He began to cry. Mr. Demarco has never touched anybody's heart. When he cries people wait until he stops, or they change the subject.

"He hides. My brother hides," he said. "He won't come out. He says that everybody is out to get him. They want to poison him. They are spying on him. But nobody believes him. It is awful. Do you mean to tell me that there is no hope, no cure, for somebody like that? They call him a paranoid schizophrenic. What good is a name when my brother is scared, and alone? All you did last time was get four cops and two psychiatrists and jump on my brother and send him to the hospital. Then they dumped all that stupid medicine in him and sent him home worse off than ever . . ." He paused. He didn't know what to do with his hands.

"You guys are getting paid. Thirty, forty thousand a year. These mental places cost millions to run and you don't have any way of helping my brother? Last month I spent ten days in the hospital after he beat me up. Three broken ribs." He pulled his shirt up. His sad, scrawny body revealed no bruises. "He wouldn't let me out of the house for a week. Held a knife to my throat! He told me if I called the mental health people again he'd kill me."

"Have you thought about moving out?" I said.

"Leave my brother alone? Are you telling me to abandon my brother? Anyway, if I left him he might really kill somebody. I got to keep an eye on him. He listens to me. If I don't talk sense to him, who will?"

"Mr. Demarco, this is the emergency . . ."

"See. See. The runaround. See! All of these places are alike. I suppose you are going to tell me to move out, let my brother starve. Man, he's helpless. He can't take care of himself. You guys sitting around on your fucking asses, doing nothing, right? Pulling down forty, fifty thou a year, not curing anybody . . ."

"Listen, Mr. Demarco," I said, "I have work to do. I don't have any answers for you. None. If you want us to pick up your brother, we could consider that. Make a complaint and we will decide whether to come out again or not. Is he a danger to himself or others?"

"I've been telling you he's a danger. He might stab some innocent person who walks up to the front door and says hello. Are you going to sit there and do nothing about that? Let him kill an innocent person? You make me sore. You know, I could bomb this place. I'm that mad. I could get a machine gun and mow down you fuckers. That's what."

"Mr. Demarco, cut out that crap."

"I'm sore. I think how alone my brother is. Nobody cares in the world. My brother thinks they are poisoning him again. He's helpless. All we get is the runaround. I could kill somebody, I get so angry. Can't you do something?"

"Mr. Demarco, that is crazy talk. Maybe we ought to evaluate you . . ."

"Oh, no you don't! See! See how you are! Some innocent citizen walks in to get help for his brother and right away you want to put him in the nuthouse. Nobody is ever going to . . . to put me . . . in one of those places again."

"When were you hospitalized, Mr. Demarco?" I asked.

"Oh, no you don't!" he said loudly. "No you don't. I'm not here for myself, anyway. I'm here for my brother. See, I'm really concerned about my brother. I'm not like other people,

people who don't care about other people. I care, see, about my brother. He's getting where he hears those voices again."

He peered at me closely, examining my face. Did I care? I blinked and looked away.

"I got to go," he said, "before you think of locking me up. Boy, wouldn't that be something."

* *

Christmas is closing in on us. Crowds mill around the many valley shopping centers. It is warm out. Harry and I foolishly stop for lunch in a restaurant in one of the new shopping malls.

A skinny black man, distinctly out of place in white suburbia, stands beside the glass talking out loud to passers-by. Seems to think he's John Wayne. He plugs the shoppers with his two six-gun forefingers following a quick draw. Then he places the guns back in imaginary holsters. Another quick draw. Zap! I got you! Pow! You're dead. Nobody plays along, grabbing his side and saying you got me. They probably realize he means it. He shoots them again and again and they get deader and deader each time.

Harry walks over and talks to the man. He smiles and nods at Harry, looking down at the polished floor like a chastened child. He walks away. Harry does not reveal what he said to him.

31

We thought the M.P. had finally put his mother out of his mind after the last time she disowned him, but he must have some of his mother's heroic stubborness. Or maybe he just wants a mother again. Last time she hardly recognized him. But later she called him up and sounded almost sane. He got his hopes up to where he thought he might have a mother again. Then she asked to speak to his boss at the plant where he now worked. The boss's strained expression told him that Mama hadn't quite made it. She was telling him tales of her cosmic travels and of that demon who wouldn't get himself lost.

We drove to the address she gave him. It was an old, rundown shack on a vacant lot to the rear of an abandoned plumbing shop. We stumbled along through the loose dirt clods, the marine, Harry, and I, cautiously approaching the small back window. We heard heavy breathing and bed springs bouncing. I pushed the young marine back. He fought me, lunging forward as if obsessed by curiosity.

There is a crazy lady humping inside, I thought, and her son here will stand at attention while his mind blows watching Mama crazy-fucking some old wino inside this rundown shack on the last day of his life.

His chin was over my right shoulder. Poor guy couldn't help himself. He was breathing heavily, lusting to have his innocence explode right into his own mama. Harry was near tears.

"Get back," I whispered. I said it too loudly. The springs stopped jumping. We waited, terribly embarrassed, looking at dirt clods, watching the traffic roll by. I watched two handsome young valley girls, well fed and laughing, driving by in their boyfriends' cars.

The springs began their eerie squeaking again. Now heavy breathing. Grunts. Words! Words! The old wino dug sex descriptions while in the act. The son lurched off to vomit in the bushes.

Harry and I stared over the ledge into the open window. It took a minute or two to adjust to the darkened room. They were there all right, locked in sexual embrace. The skinny old lady was naked. Now I am stuck additionally and forever with this terrible, vacant look on her face. And that, Harry and I agreed, was what you would call an invasion of privacy.

Maybe we should have picked her up, but her persistence and courage were making believers out of us. She would be out of the hospital in a week anyway.

Harry and I grabbed the M.P. and headed for a bar Harry knew. He had a couple of beers but then became uncomfortable. Before leaving, he thanked us for "helping" his mother—he said it without sarcasm.

32

Christmas has arrived. There is a half-gallon jug of cheap wine in the coffee room refrigerator. It explains why Harry has been gabbing it up so much with the stenos lately. It is snowing in the East right now. The papers say that cars were skidding all over the place yesterday on the sleet-covered streets. I think of my son and his family in New York. The sharp wind off the river, dismal gray stacks on the New Jersey shore. He is probably jogging with his dog up the barren paths of the park right at this moment, sinking into the rain-sodden leaves, his head down looking for chuck holes. He will stop at Grant's Tomb and head back.

The dapper young man seated across from me has flown in from the East to have us check out his mother-in-law, who called him earlier in the day, screaming terrible obscenities coast to coast.

She is obviously insane. She has been threatening people, saying she will hurt them or kill them. She isn't paying her rent. He has to settle the situation in a hurry and fly back. He tells me proudly of his company's generosity. They flew him out here at their expense.

He looks out the big window, scanning the valley to the north.

"I was brought up in Pasadena," he says. "Went to PCC."

"Really?"

"Yeah." He surveys the office. "I was going to be a psychologist once. I was going to help people, you know. I don't know. I guess I decided making money was what I really wanted. I don't know."

"It's a good field," I say.

"I couldn't handle all that behavioral crap."

"Me neither."

"My mother-in-law is something else," he says. "I probably should have given her a Rorschach or something before I got married. You know, you really ought to check out your wife's parents."

I agree it wouldn't be a bad idea.

"She was always so tough, you know. Frankly, she scares the crap out of me."

He grins. "She scares my wife too. The old bitch is really something. And she is a sex fiend. Down deep, I mean. God, is she a sex fiend. Really."

"She represses it, probably."

"Boy, talk about projection. That old lady *invented* projection. Oh, *she* isn't a sex fiend. Not *her.* No, sir, not her. *You.* You're the sex fiend."

"I didn't know it showed."

He smiles. "You know what I mean." He makes a teeter-totter gesture. "Frankly, I think the old gal is a little . . . a dyke, I think. Of course, it's *you* that's all sexually screwed up. Not her." He catches himself. He blushes slightly. "You know . . . Would you believe, she even accused me . . ." He gulps. "She has even accused me of balling her. Can you imagine that? I mean, me balling my own mother-in-law."

"It's happened before," I say.

"Sure, I know, but I wouldn't do anything like that. That would be so dumb, for one thing . . ."

Especially, I think, if the lady goes crazy. Then it is all kiss and tell.

We meet thc young man at his mother-in-law's motel.

Harry maneuvers the big gray wagon through a thick, sand-colored archway into a large parking area. The tires growl softly on the gravel.

We ring the bell. There is a rattle of chains and locks. A face peeks out. "Yes?"

"It's me, Marie."

"Who? Who are you? What do you want?"

"It's me, Marie. Brad."

"Brad? Oh, Brad. Sure, Brad. So what do you want?"

"Jesus, Marie, I haven't seen you in months. Is that any kind of greeting for your son-in-law? I want to say hello and my friends here want to come in for a chat."

"I thought you were away. I thought you had gone somewhere. Who are these men?"

"I live back East, you know that. I live with your daughter."

"Who? That tramp? Come right on in, gentlemen. Come right on in. Boy, Marilee is no daughter, Brad." She guffaws. "She's a whore. You know that."

"Come on, Marie. Don't talk like that."

"Whore," she mutters, like a little kid sneaking in the last word. "Whore."

Harry appraises her. She is a large, muscular woman. Formidable. He glances at me meaningfully. As we enter the front room he takes a strategic position at the dining table behind her.

She turns to face him. "What do you men want?"

I hand her my card. "Brad, what is this?" She pushes her chin into his face. He looks down and away like a small boy ashamed of his naughty behavior. She follows his face with her own, intimately leaning toward him. "What have you *done,* Brad? What are you doing to me?"

Brad takes hold. "These men are here to talk to you, Marie. You've been threatening people."

"Me? Threatening people? Now isn't that something?" She looks upward, addressing the ceiling. "Isn't that something? And who told you that, Brad?"

As I write this I relive the fear of this morning's call, and I am aware that my enthusiasm for these PET adventures, let alone my willingness to participate, is rapidly waning. It is not the same. I look over at Harry's desk. It is occupied by Phil, a well-intentioned but inexperienced young man. Harry is off duty.

It began as a quiet, noneventful PET Friday until the young woman telephoned. It was her husband, she said. He was losing contact with reality again. Again? Yes, he had been hospitalized previously. What was his present behavior? He was seeing the devil again, she said. Another possession case. I am afraid of him, she said. He sees the devil in me and in the children. Even in the cat. The cat was missing. Had he tried to exorcise the devil, perhaps?

She spoke in a flat voice. The many years of anxiety, living with a borderline psychotic individual, had taken their toll. His disturbance had killed her love. She remained with him out of duty. Where was she at this moment? In a motel. Could she meet us at the house? Of course.

Was he a big man? He was six-foot three and weighed about two hundred and forty pounds. Two forty? Yes. Any weapons? Guns? No, she said, only the kitchen utensils, knives and all that. She doubted that he would use them. Just before she hung up she added that it had taken nine men to subdue him the last time. *Nine* men?

These anxious questions drew laughter from the gathering. The administrative assistant asked me if I had my medical insurance up to date.

I had forgotten to obtain the woman's home address. Fortunately I had her telephone number. I tried, sneakily, to dial her back and pretend that I needed more information. The social work intern caught me asking her for the address.

"Boy, are you nervous!" he said loudly. "Forgot to get the address, eh?"

The group roared with laughter. A new staff member joined in the fun. Look at how his feet are fidgeting, he said laughing gleefully. No respect, I said. No respect for us old guys.

I began coordinating the PET action. "We will need eight people. We will need four policemen, two ambulance attendants—that makes six. Oh, yes, Phil and myself, the two of us . . ."

"You could stay here at the clinic and coordinate it from here," the administrative assistant said.

"Why don't you come along?" I said. "We could use you."

"No siree," he said. "There is a full moon tonight."

"Tell the police we don't want an entire army there," I told Phil. "And no helicopters. And tell the ambulance people not to use the siren."

We met the young man's disheveled wife at a street corner nearby. She was a small, pretty woman, more practical than cold.

"Well," I said, "here we are." The police pulled up. I introduced Phil and myself to the one who appeared to be the leader. He seemed preoccupied. Inexplicably, he walked off. I tried another officer. He listened and then translated the situation to the other three. They retired to the back seat of a squad car.

"It is going to be one of those leaderless jobs," I mumbled to Phil. "These guys won't follow our orders." I showed an officer my PET card. He hadn't asked for identification, but now he examined it intently. He checked my face carefully against the picture, looking down and up again. He wouldn't let go of it. Finally I wrenched it away. He looked at me angrily, as if he wanted to arrest me.

"Where's your ID?" I asked Phil.

"I never got one."

"You don't have any *identification* after all this time?"

He shook his head.

"And nobody has ever *asked* for it?"

He nodded. "I have my county business cards," he said.

I instructed the policemen. The woman would let us into

the house. They would lead the way in and I would then evaluate the man. We were to use force only if he attacked us. They nodded uncomprehendingly. One officer smacked a closed fist into his other hand.

The woman led the six of us to her house. We walked single file. The policemen trailed to the rear. I gestured to them to hurry up. They ignored me. It was all wrong already. A crowd was gathering. The man inside could see us coming. I was getting tense.

No one would approach the front door. "You guys . . ." I said. No response. "You . . ." The young woman walked up and tried the screen door. It was locked. I followed her. Phil walked behind me. She knocked.

Her husband opened the door a few inches, peeking out.

"Harold," she said. "These men . . ." She did not know what to say.

Nor did I. "I'm Dr. Crain, Mr. Johnson. I would like to . . ."

He eyed the policemen standing in full view on the lawn. "No," he said. "No."

"Harold," she said. "Please."

"I would like to talk to you, Mr. Johnson." I showed him my card.

He looked away. "No," he said. "I would rather not." He smiled knowingly. "That's all right," he added. "I really would rather not. You see, there is evil everywhere, and no, I really would rather not . . ."

He slammed the door shut. I looked around. What to do? I looked at Phil. He looked at me. "We can't force our way in," I said.

"Why not?" a policeman said. "We can break the door down if his wife tells us to."

"I don't want . . ." I could not decide what to do. He was psychotic, I was certain of that. Possession by the devil was becoming a more common psychotic symptom. But it didn't make sense to break into his house like that.

I paced the porch for a moment. Everyone watched me. Suddenly I was the chief and I would give the orders. And of course I would have to lead the charge. The police shuffled about.

"Well, let's go on in," I said. No movement. "To hell with it," I said to Phil. "Let's go back to the clinic. Let's call it off. I don't *know* he is psychotic at this moment. We can't break in." I explained this to the wife and the officer standing next to me. We would simply have to let the man determine the next move.

She moaned. "No," she said. "Please. He won't . . ."

A young, grim-faced policeman said loudly, *"This man has barricaded himself in there, and . . ."*

Jesus! Suddenly this home visit was taking off before our eyes. They were thinking of open warfare, and tear gas.

"Look," I said to the woman. "Let's tear the screen and unlatch the screen door." We tried it. I cut my finger. The latch wouldn't give. As I fiddled with the latch I sensed the man's presence against the door inside, not four inches from me. He was hearing all this. Waves of terror hit me. *What if he had a gun?* Wives liked to leave that out when reporting or asking for help. I wondered how many people we visit might just finger the trigger and then decide not to pull it—and how many policemen carry ghostly scars of death imagined.

Suddenly the wife walked up and ripped the screen door off one hinge. She pulled her key out of her purse and opened the front door.

She pushed the door open and walked in. He looked at her as if she were a stranger. I placed my foot against the door and readied myself for the blow I was certain was coming. I waved my hand behind my back, signaling the officers to come into the house. No one moved. Finally a young policeman slipped by me into the room.

"No," the man said. "No, I would rather not." He began to breathe deeply. He inhaled and exhaled loudly, throwing his chest out like an animal, making a fierce expression to frighten me. I smiled. This was my territory now. Two more policemen slid between us into the room. They stood in a small circle some eight or ten feet back.

"Is this America?" he yelled suddenly. "Is this the United States of America?" I followed his eyes to the four blue-clothed policemen standing in the living room of his home.

"The Lord will punish you!" he screamed, startling us.

"Do not invoke the name of the Lord," a young officer said. "Not in that way."

The man turned to the officer and smiled. He quoted a sentence from the Bible regarding the Lord's vengeance. The officer topped him with a quote regarding the Lord's gentleness and forgiving nature. The man smiled again. He is a gentle man, I thought, underneath it all.

I worked at convincing him he should go to the hospital voluntarily. We would have him lie down on the gurney. Let us strap him down. Don't fight it. He would be out of the hospital in no time. "Maybe in a week," I said. "Come on, let's see you go voluntarily."

"No," he said, "I would rather not."

"I know you have lost your job and haven't been able to get another one," I said. "And you know you are losing contact. You know that from before. You went through all this before."

He dropped his head. He was sane for a moment. He nodded. Then he looked up into my eyes questioningly.

"That's right," I said. "Look into my eyes and see if I mean you any harm." He glanced at me and then looked away. The deep breathing began again. He pumped his chest up, then exhaled loudly. Whoosh! Whoosh! He was working himself up. When would he strike out?

I caught the officers' eyes, gesturing for them to grab him. No one moved. More talk. Whoosh! Whoosh! It was getting eerie. Suddenly he shouted a frightening animal scream. I jumped. No one moved.

He smiled, aware of some inner power now. He spoke in

a loud staccato. "In—a minute—from—now—I am—going—to make—you—get—out." He paused. *"Get out of my house!"* He swept his hand to the door. It was a gesture of his omnipotent powers, his magical godlike abilities.

I blinked. For a second I found myself transported through the screen and out onto the porch. He seemed puzzled, momentarily. He examined his hand like a shortstop looking for the hole in his glove after an error.

"Argh! Argh! Argh!" he screamed, moving toward the officers.

They piled on, flaying away, grabbing and leaning and shoving and weighing him down with their bodies as he struggled mightily, lost inside this blue, multilimbed, enraged creature. I looked on. Sunglasses shot by my head. I was shocked yet calm, fascinated at the immense pleasure these tough kids were showing, these four bullies loving the *feel* of all this violent thrashing about. I too had felt the thrill of it before.

Six more officers ran into the room. Reinforcements had been summoned. They were waved away. There was no room to grab anything. Phil looked at me. Sure enough, a helicopter could be heard overhead. Then three tall men in civilian clothes entered the room. Police officials. They observed the scene calmly.

The patient had long since crumpled into submission and had gone further than that, much further: he had curled into the position before his birth—and then he was gone. It seemed strangely unnecessary to put the restraints on his arms and legs.

The policemen stood up one at a time. They looked down in wonderment at his still body. His breathing was soft and easy like an infant's. Gently they placed his large, bound body onto the gurney.

I began filling out the papers.

Reason for hospitalization: "He was delusional and hallucinatory, also violent. Ten police officers were required to subdue him." I underlined the word *ten*. Then I tore it up and wrote, "Ten police officers were summoned, along with a helicopter and three police lieutenants." It would impress them up at Camarillo.

The room was empty now. The wife had left earlier. Someone said she was next door at a neighbor's. The man's wallet was on the couch. I placed it out of sight under a shirt. Before I closed the door I looked around the room. It was a lonely room and strangely quiet. I could feel the young man's gentle presence. His coat was draped over a chair at the table in the dining room, as if he had turned his back to me. I closed the door.

34

Harry has been taking his sick leave and his unused vacation time. He hasn't said so, but I am sure now he will be leaving soon. He seems preoccupied and distant. Probably it is his new business deal. He doesn't say. We stopped for a beer the other day and it was the same old Harry again. We talked about the interesting calls we had been on together. We were like two old soldiers meeting after the war. We both realized then that the partnership was seeing its last days. We didn't speak of it. He said he thought Phil was working out all right, though he had a lot to learn. It was as if he were deeding him to me as his replacement. I said there was nobody who gave us all the feeling of security that he did. When wrestling was called for, Harry, you were the man, I said. We both noticed my use of the past tense but we didn't mention it.

*   *

Phil handed me a telephone inquiry card. A mother of a young woman claimed her daughter was seeing things that weren't there. A baby sitting on a potty chair, for example.

"Is this a valid call?" he asked. "It doesn't sound like an emergency, just seeing things."

"She might be regressing," I said. "We better take a look."

"Her mother impressed me as being a real bitch," Phil said. "It was her tone of voice. You know, you get so you can figure people out just from their telephone conversation, can't you? She said her daughter had kicked her out of her apartment, her own mother."

We knocked on the door. A heavy, homely girl greeted us brightly. She stared at us with a wide, inappropriate smile. "Hello there, you guys," she said. "Come on in." I had the urge to tell her not to let strangers in like that.

I handed the girl my card, which she didn't read. She placed it against her breast. She smoothed her skirt like a middle-aged matron. She sat down on the couch, patting a place next to her. We sat in chairs opposite. The smile remained fixed on her face. She was obviously not starving, considering how heavy she was. There were open boxes of crackers on the kitchen sink. Crackers were strewn all about.

"How are you?" she asked, as if we were old friends.

Her question referred to another place, another time. We were two members of an audience who had walked backstage while the show was on. How come these people were getting to look so familiar?

Her eyes darted around the room. "Listen," she said excitedly, "do you hear?"

"What did she hear?" Phil asked me in a whisper.

"Isn't that sweet?" Her expression was oddly beautiful, serene.

"Yes," I said. "It really is. What is it?"

"You know," she said. "Come."

I nodded at Phil. She placed her arm under his confidently.

She led him toward the bedroom. He looked at me. I followed them. She dropped his arm at the doorway. We stood there, the three of us. There was a whispery, angelic aura to the girl, as if she had been mysteriously redeemed by this madness of hers, the terrible dues of it.

She approached a small wooden potty chair. She spoke softly, insistently, to the baby there, the presence unseen by us. She turned, flushed and radiant.

"Isn't she darling?" she said.

"Yes," I said.

We called her mother to let her know we had hospitalized her daughter. We learned she had had a recent abortion, which caused the break. It was her boyfriend's fault, she said. Her first and only love, who left her when he learned she was pregnant. Naturally.

It was right out of Peyton Place. Her mother spoke in a flat, dead tone of voice. "Just like a man," she intoned. "I told her that men were no damn good. I told her. All they want is one thing. And look where it got her. I told her that men were no damn good."

Yes, lady. You told her that for years. You told her that sex, loving a man, was something nasty. You never let her become a full-blown woman. So now she has dreamed up a second chance in that invisible baby sitting there on the potty chair.

35

It's not the same here with Harry gone. He simply did not show up for work one morning. Word has it that he skipped town. He could have said good-by. I'm saddened and disappointed that he left that way. I check my mail each morning but I come up empty.

It is as if he were never here. Strangely, he seems to have taken his spirit and presence with him, leaving us a single, dim memory of himself.

Just too much scooping, Harry? The kid with the bloody feet, maybe? Or the M.P.'s mother, humping away with that wild, empty look in her eyes in that ratty old shack? No. Old Harry is off chasing a dream somewhere.

So now I have this inexperienced kid with a good heart on the PET team, and here we go again, chasing the M.P.'s mother down the street and behind this market, tromping over fucking cardboard boxes. She is screaming, "May God rebuke you! May God rebuke you!" I wish she wouldn't yell that. She is practically falling over backward, pointing that long, bony finger in my face. Her arms must be ten yards long. How does she run so fast backward?

Phil is panting hard behind me. He is in surprisingly lousy shape for a one-time phys ed major. His knees are buckling and going in two directions at once. I swear he has no idea what he is doing here chasing this old lady who's running for her right to be crazy and starve to death and sleep with old winos.

Phil is wrestling her to the ground now, holding her tight and mean-faced, with his teeth grinding like he wants to kill all the world's craziness forever. Poor kid is crying while she is screaming "May God rebuke you!" right into his ear at close range. It will ring in there for months.

"Crazy lady," I say, "you win. You *win.* Shit." She smiles at me. We are old friends now.

* *

These are the wayfarers, society's losers. Everyman. They are joined on occasion by presidents and other notables, but mostly they are just people. All they really want is love and acceptance. Is that so hard to give?

They are off by the side of the road now. They can't make that necessary adjustment, can't find that tenuous, fragile balance between their inner worlds and the outside world, with all its crazy messages and its preoccupation with everything but what is necessary for life. So they drift off into that last space where one can hide—the human mind.

And they close the door.